Getting Pregnant
the Natural Way

the women's 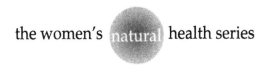 health series

Getting Pregnant
the Natural Way

Deborah Gordon, M.D., Series Editor

D. S. FEINGOLD
AND
DEBORAH GORDON, M.D.

A Lynn Sonberg Book

JOHN WILEY & SONS, INC.
New York · Chichester · Weinheim · Brisbane · Singapore · Toronto

Published by John Wiley & Sons, Inc.
Published simultaneously in Canada

Illustrations by Jackie Aher

Design and production by Navta Associates, Inc.

This publication is designed to provide accurate and authoritative information in regard to the subject matter covered. It is sold with the understanding that the publisher is not engaged in rendering professional services. If professional advice or other expert assistance is required, the services of a competent professional person should be sought.

Library of Congress Cataloging-in-Publication Data

Gordon, Deborah (Deborah R.)
    Getting Pregnant the natural way / D. S. Feingold, Deborah Gordon.
    p. cm. — (The women's natural health series)
    Includes index.
    ISBN 13: 978-1-62045-703-0
    1. Pregnancy—Complications—Alternative treatment. 2. Infertility—Complications—Alternative treatment. 3. Alternative medicine. 4. Naturopathy. I. Feingold, David S., 1922– II. Title. III. Series.

RC889 .G66 2000
618.1'7806—dc21   00-035908

10 9 8 7 6 5 4 3 2 1

Important Note

This book is for informational purposes only. It is not intended to take the place of medical advice from a trained medical professional. Readers are advised to consult a physician or other qualified health professional regarding treatment of all of their health problems or before acting on any of the information or advice in this book.

This book is intended to provide selected information about infertility. Research about male and female infertility is ongoing and subject to conflicting interpretations. As a result, there is no guarantee that what we know about this subject won't change with time.

Contents

Getting Pregnant
the Natural Way

Introduction:
The Path to Fertility

By Deborah Gordon, M.D.

It's a familiar scenario: after establishing careers and settling down, a couple in their mid-30s decides to have a child. Six months pass, then a year, but the woman is still not pregnant. Friends and family offer advice, articles and books are consulted, and eventually a doctor's appointment is made. Tests are done, followed perhaps by a series of drug treatments and surgical procedures. What was supposed to be a joyful process turns into an ordeal marked by anxiety, frustration, depression, and possibly physical discomfort.

As a medical doctor and classical homeopath, I have witnessed firsthand the trials and tribulations of patients facing infertility. All health problems cause distress, of course, but the inability to get pregnant is one of the most traumatic experiences a woman can endure.

It's hard to pinpoint an exact moment when infertility became a household word. But there's no doubt that recently we've been made more aware that many couples have trouble conceiving a child. The issue seems to be everywhere—on TV talk shows, magazine covers, books, radio, the Internet. It seems as if the media is presenting the struggle to get pregnant as the norm and trouble-free conception as the exception.

In fact, there has been only a slight rise in infertility in the last few decades. The greatest single factor in this upturn is the trend to start families much later in life than in the past. Since fertility declines with age, particularly for women, couples trying to conceive in their 30s and 40s are more likely to encounter difficulties. The dramatic increase in sexually transmitted diseases has played a significant role in reproductive problems, and many scientific researchers believe that the proliferation of environmental toxins has also taken its toll on fertility.

Even if infertility is not spiraling out of control, it is a very real concern for a lot of people. Each year, more than a million North Americans pursue treatment for infertility. The majority consult conventional doctors, who do an infertility workup and then, depending on the diagnosis, usually recommend drugs and/or high-tech procedures such as in vitro fertilization.

Since the 1980s, great strides have been made in reproductive medicine. Thanks to a vast amount of research, physicians now understand far more about how conception occurs and what can prevent it from happening. These advances have led to a boom in assisted reproductive technology, or ART. In addition to in vitro fertilization, a range of options are now available, including gamete intrafallopian transfer (GIFT), zygote intrafallopian transfer (ZIFT), egg donation, and gestational carriers, among others. Intrauterine insemination (IUI) is another possibility, as is surrogate pregnancy.

Unfortunately, despite the progress in understanding and treating infertility, only a minority of women who undergo high-tech procedures ultimately achieve the goal of pregnancy. Although statistics differ, it appears that the success rate is about 20%. Thus, four out of five couples are left still wanting a child.

In recent years, more and more people have been turning to alternative or complementary medicine for answers to their health problems. Whereas small numbers of North Americans have long sought out holistic practitioners, the '90s into the 21st century have witnessed a phenomenal explosion in the use of herbal remedies, acupuncture, homeopathy, chiropractic medicine, mind/body medicine, and a host of other therapies. These approaches are no longer hidden alternatives to conventional medicine but rather well-respected and well-researched treatment options that enhance health. Complementary medicine is now widely used for everything from colds and the flu to chronic fatigue syndrome to hypertension.

The application of natural medicine to infertility dates back thousands of years. Yet only in the last decade or so have a substantial amount of people begun to pursue alternative treatments to improve their chances of conception.

If you are trying to have a child, there are several compelling reasons to explore alternative therapies. First and foremost, based on the clinical experience of hundreds of practitioners, these techniques can help you get pregnant. This is not to say that alternative health care offers some miracle cure; neither mainstream nor alternative medicine can promise a pregnancy. But infertility is a complex condition often caused by a multitude of chronic factors, and many of these respond to natural remedies. For example, hormonal problems are one of the main culprits in delaying conception. By altering diet, taking nutritional supplements, using herbs, and practicing relaxation exercises, many women are able to restore hormonal balance and eventually get pregnant.

Second, in addition to improving your fertility, alternative treatments will enhance your overall health. Indeed, these two outcomes are closely linked: in general, the better your health, the more likely you are to conceive. Consider the fact that many of the greatest health risks—smoking, drinking, drug use, obesity, poor diet, stress—pose the biggest threat to fertility. By changing your lifestyle and supporting these changes with natural remedies, you will enjoy a higher level of physical vitality.

Third, alternative therapies can give you more control over one of the most emotional medical issues anyone can face. While practitioners play an essential role in natural medicine, self-care is just as important. By forming a positive partnership with your physician based on mutual respect and responsibility, you and your partner can face the challenges of infertility with greater confidence and less anxiety.

Choosing a course of treatment for infertility is an incredibly personal decision. Some women who have difficulty getting pregnant are not interested in pursuing in vitro fertilization or taking another woman's egg into their body. Others are prepared to do anything to have a child.

This book offers many ideas for people in both categories. If you want to follow a natural conception program, the one described here will provide an excellent start. If you have tried, are currently using, or are considering fertility drugs and high-tech procedures, many of the steps described here will also be helpful. Indeed, natural methods of enhancing fertility can complement conventional infertility treatment, giving you the greatest possible range of choices.

As a family physician practicing complementary medicine, I have seen patients make incredible improvements in their health through holistic therapies. By changing their diet, exercising regularly, using herbs and nutritional supplements, and decreasing stress, they have regained vitality, which in turn has allowed them to get pregnant.

I believe very strongly that parenting starts long before the baby is born, even before conception. I love to meet with both parents before conception to lay the healthiest and most fertile ground for the new life they are planning to create. I encourage partners to look carefully at their own life and make positive changes that will be of benefit both now and in the future.

This is a perfect time to take the steps necessary to enhance your physical and emotional well-being. By preparing for a successful, healthy pregnancy, you will also be planting the seeds for healthy children guided by loving, vital parents.

CHAPTER ONE

What Is Infertility?

Nearly every woman remembers her early days of being sexually active, when she lived in fear that any and all sexual experiences would result in pregnancy. It comes as a shock to find out later that conception can be difficult.

The truth is that human reproduction is an incredibly sensitive process that can be thrown off by many forces. So while it's natural to feel frustrated if you're having a hard time getting pregnant, you should know that fertility problems are both very common and in many cases reversible.

The first step is to educate yourself. As you'll see, infertility is a complex condition often caused by multiple factors. The more you understand, the better you'll be able to decide on a course of treatment.

This chapter defines infertility and outlines the various causes that can affect both women and men, from stress to environmental toxins, from nutritional deficiencies to sexual dysfunction. We set the record straight on some of the myths about infertility, including the notion that it's strictly a question of hormones, eggs, and sperm. And we discuss how fertility is inextricably linked to your overall physical and emotional health, as well as that of your partner.

The Facts about Infertility

The word *infertility* is commonly used, but little care is taken to define what it is—and what it isn't. Stated simply, infertility is the inability to get pregnant or carry a pregnancy to term. A diagnosis of infertility is generally made if, after 12 months of regular, unprotected intercourse (or insemination), conception hasn't occurred. Infertility also applies if a woman repeatedly conceives but can't maintain a pregnancy. Within medical circles, the words *impaired fecundity* are often used interchangeably with infertility. The term *subfertile* has a slightly different meaning, referring to the reduced fertility of women as they enter their late 30s.

Infertility, impaired fecundity, and subfertility should not be confused with *sterility*, which means that conception is impossible under any circumstances. Unless you've been told for a fact that you or your partner is sterile as a result of bilateral oophorectomy (surgical removal of both ovaries) or as a possible side effect of medical treatments such as chemotherapy and radiation therapy, you probably won't know that you have a fertility problem until you start trying to get pregnant.

Primary Versus Secondary Infertility

There are two basic types of infertility: primary and secondary. Primary infertility is diagnosed if a woman has never been pregnant and has not conceived after 12 months of regular intercourse. Secondary infertility applies if a woman has been pregnant before but is having trouble conceiving again.

As discussed in this chapter, it's important to remember with both kinds of infertility that the problem may be with either the man or the woman. In some situations, both partners contribute to conception difficulties.

KNOWLEDGE AND ACTION: THE FIRST STEPS TO BETTER HEALTH

As with any medical condition, educating yourself is one of the keys to enhancing your fertility. Becoming familiar with the basics of reproduction and the wide variety of both alternative and conventional treatments will relieve some of the fear and powerlessness that go along with infertility. You'll also be able to make more informed choices about treatment that take into account not only the question of pregnancy but your overall health and well-being.

While there's no reason to panic if you're having trouble conceiving, it makes sense to take control of the situation. Many couples have a hard time admitting that they have a fertility problem. After each attempt, they tell themselves that maybe they will conceive the next time. Rushing to the doctor after 1 or 2 months is premature, but if pregnancy hasn't occurred within 6 months or so of concerted effort, it's time to take stock of the situation. Focusing on the information in this book and/or consulting a professional are options. If you are over 30 years old and have a history of pelvic inflammatory infection, endometriosis, painful periods, miscarriage, or irregular menstrual cycles, you may want to seek help sooner. The same is true if you know that your partner has a low sperm count or other related condition.

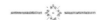

Factors That Affect Fertility

"Infertility is never a completely straightforward affair," says Christiane Northrup, M.D., author of *Women's Bodies, Women's*

Wisdom and a leading authority on women's health. Roughly one in five cases of infertility cannot be traced to any known medical condition. However, many women who have been told they are infertile due to a specific physical problem get pregnant without any treatment.

According to Dr. Northrup, the most common reasons for infertility are:

- Irregular ovulation
- Endometriosis
- History of pelvic infection from an intrauterine device (IUD) or other source, causing scarring of the fallopian tubes
- Stress
- Immune system problems
- Low sperm counts

In Chapter 2, we'll look closely at the menstrual cycle and the female reproductive system, examining what facilitates conception and what can prevent it. Chapter 3 will discuss male fertility factors. Here we consider some of the broader issues that affect fertility.

Age

The dramatic trend toward delaying childbearing is perhaps the single greatest factor contributing to infertility. The older a woman is before having her first child, the greater the risk that she will have trouble conceiving and/or carrying a pregnancy to term.

"In the modern world where women have to go out and work, they tend to put off having children until much later," says Daoshing Ni, L.Ac., D.O.M., Ph.D., of Santa Monica, California. In the past, a woman might have had fewer than 40 menstrual cycles before pregnancy, whereas now there might be 12 years of monthly periods before a woman decides to have a child.

"Unfortunately, [delaying pregnancy] is an epidemic in this country," states Dr. Ni. "When that occurs, it creates several problems. First, [women's] bodies may not be in great health when they are ready to have a child, and it may be difficult for them to get pregnant. Sometimes their hormones may be out of balance and they may already have fibroids or endometriosis problems, which further inhibits them from getting pregnant."

There are many reasons why couples are waiting to have children. For women, the sexual revolution of the 1960s and 1970s led to unprecedented freedoms, both in their personal and professional lives. The availability of cheap, reliable contraceptives allowed women to enjoy a new level of sexual liberty without the overriding fear of an unwanted pregnancy. At the same time, the idea of women pursuing full-fledged careers became accepted.

The effect of these two transformative social developments was to change the way both men and women approached the issue of parenting. Instead of marrying and starting a family in their 20s, millions of people put off such commitments until their 30s. This shift in priorities continues today, with many women trying to become pregnant for the first time at age 35 or older.

Although many doctors will counsel their patients that they can have a baby anytime—certainly well into their 40s—this advice can be very misleading. A woman has an excellent chance of conceiving throughout her 20s, and though fertility begins to decline after age 30, prospects for conception are still good in the absence of serious problems. Most experts agree, however, that a woman's fertility drops sharply after age 35, so by her late 30s she is about 30% less fertile than in her early 20s. At age 40 and beyond, pregnancy attempts are frequently unsuccessful and require a greater degree of medical intervention.

Although more and more women are conceiving and giving birth in their late 30s and 40s, many of these babies are the result of assisted reproductive technology (ART) procedures such as in vitro fertilization and egg donation. These techniques do work for some women, but there are physical, emotional, and monetary prices. And in many cases, they do not lead to the birth of a child, leaving couples financially depleted and psychologically drained.

Environment

Although rarely discussed by conventional fertility specialists, environmental contaminants are considered by many leading alternative practitioners and researchers to pose a serious threat to procreation. New studies have raised troubling questions about how reproduction is affected by pesticides, hormones, household chemicals, and air and water pollution. "Conditions on this earth may not favor fertility the way they used to," explains Dr. Northrup. "Humans cannot pollute and overcrowd this planet without consequences to our bodies, and infertility is one of them."

Nutrition

Every aspect of human health is impacted by what we eat, and fertility is no exception. Few of us get the nutrients we need from our diet. On the contrary, we may fill our plates with high-fat, high-sugar, low-fiber foods. These consumption habits do little to maintain our reproductive systems, and in fact can compromise fertility. In Chapter 6, we'll discuss how good nutrition, along with supplementation, can pave the way to a healthy pregnancy.

Digestion and Elimination

In many alternative healing traditions, the digestion and elimination organs are regarded as central to reproduction. Without proper digestion, the body doesn't get the nutrition it needs to support conception and pregnancy. And if wastes aren't eliminated efficiently, the resulting buildup of toxins can lead to infections and other conditions that may compromise fertility. These issues will also be covered in Chapter 6.

Weight

Obesity is on the rise and the health implications are grave. One of the best-documented effects is the disruption of normal menstrual and hormonal function, which can lead directly to infertility. In contrast, inadequate body fat can also interfere with the menstrual cycle and hormonal balance, producing the same results. Women with eating disorders have a disproportionately high rate of infertility, as do some female athletes such as long-distance runners. Chapter 6 will explore the weight issue in more detail.

Caffeine, Alcohol, Tobacco, and Drug Use

These stimulants are all associated with a drop in fertility. In the case of caffeine and alcohol, small amounts may not pose much of a threat, but the safety threshold is very low. Tobacco and drugs in even tiny doses can jeopardize the chances of getting pregnant as well as having a healthy baby, as Chapter 6 will discuss.

Thyroid Problems

Thyroid dysfunction is a major factor in infertility. An underactive thyroid gland can result in hormonal imbalances, which in turn may block conception or lead to miscarriage. Thyroid disorders will be addressed in several chapters.

Sexual Dysfunction

A variety of conditions ranging from sexually transmitted diseases to excessive masturbation by men can prevent conception.

The same is true of infrequent intercourse. These issues will be considered in several chapters.

Stress and Depression

Alternative physicians believe that stress, anxiety, and depression can have a significant negative effect on conception. Recent studies have confirmed this conviction, showing a correlation between successful treatment of mood disorders and increased pregnancy. Chapter 9 will look at how stress affects fertility and describe various mind/body relaxation techniques.

Fertility Myths

Like many complex medical conditions, infertility is often misunderstood by the public. And as with most health care issues, there are differing views among conventional caregivers and alternative practitioners. Here are a few of the popular misperceptions about infertility, as well as several misguided claims sometimes supported by the fertility industry.

It's a Woman's Problem

One of the most common myths is that infertility is a woman's problem. According to the Resolve organization, the country's largest infertility association, the male-female split is about the same. Approximately 40% of infertility cases are due to female factors and another 40% to male factors; the remaining 20% either result from a combination of male and female factors or are unexplained. These numbers offer indisputable proof that both the man and the woman should be evaluated when infertility is suspected.

Low sperm count and poor motility are the most common causes of male infertility (see Chapter 3 for a thorough discussion of male factors). These sperm problems are associated with a wide range of conditions, from congenital diseases to stress and depression to sexual dysfunction.

Abortion Equals Infertility

Another popular fallacy is that if a woman has had an abortion, she can never have a baby. In reality, an uncomplicated abortion poses no long-term health risks. If the procedure was done professionally within the first trimester, a woman will probably be able to conceive and carry a baby to term in the future. However, women who suffered complications or had the procedure performed later in the pregnancy may have scar tissue that could cause fertility complications. If these circumstances apply, consult your doctor.

Hormones Are Everything

Although most physicians describe infertility as a physical condition, there is growing evidence that emotional and psychological health play a key role in the ability to conceive. Until recently, most conventional practitioners agreed that stress was simply a by-product of infertility, not a cause. This is where most holistic practitioners part company with their mainstream counterparts.

Although many medical doctors are starting to acknowledge the influence of emotional factors on fertility, frequently allopathic medicine still gives short shrift to such concerns. "The conventional management of infertility focuses on the body as a hormonal machine and in large part ignores emotional, psychological and even nutritional factors that have physical and hormonal manifestations," comments Dr. Northrup. "Many infertile women are working 60 to 80 hours per week, and are exhausted. Then they pursue having a child as though they were writing a Ph.D. dissertation. Conceiving a child is a receptive act, not a marathon event that can be programmed into your DayTimer. Several studies have indicated that excessive focus on the goal of having a child may result in premature maturation of the eggs in the ovary and subsequent release of eggs that are not ready for fertilization!"

Mind/body medicine offers a range of techniques that can help you to relax and revitalize. Such practices can prove invaluable not only in enhancing fertility but also in maintaining or restoring emotional balance.

Science Can Guarantee You a Baby

Roughly $1 billion is spent annually on attempts to overcome infertility. As we discussed in the Introduction, Western medicine has developed a variety of tests, drugs, and high-tech procedures to aid in the reproductive process. Yet despite all the advances, the majority of people who seek out these options do not end up pregnant. This does not mean that conventional approaches are ineffective, or that you should rule them out. But it does provide some perspective to balance the hype about miracle babies.

The Big Picture

Every couple's experience is somewhat different when it comes to infertility. Regardless of the particulars, it's essential that both partners be involved in the process. As we noted before, the cause may rest with the man, the woman, or both. Actively including both parties will keep one partner from feeling left out, or the other from feeling as though the entire burden of resolving the problem rests with him or her.

Remember that this journey isn't only about sperm counts and hormone levels. There is a profound emotional dimension to the experience, and often a spiritual one as well. Take the opportunity to learn as much as you can about yourself and your partner, and to build a closer relationship. If you do, your lives will be enriched regardless of the outcome.

CHAPTER TWO

The Menstrual Cycle—
What Really Happens and
What Can Go Wrong

Almost nothing is taboo anymore when it comes to sex. Sexually explicit movies, web sites, books, and magazines have proliferated beyond what anyone could have imagined a generation ago.

In this environment, you might think that most people would be well informed about how human reproduction works. Yet it is a surprising contradiction that people understand far more about sexual activity than they do about the by-product of sexual activity.

It's easy to see why. Sex education remains controversial. As a result, most youth learn little about reproduction in school. The same is true in the home, where despite the sexual revolution, apprehension about sex often keeps parents from discussing the subject with their kids. Those parents who do want to educate their children may themselves be hampered by insufficient knowledge or resources. The consequences are epidemics of unwanted teenage pregnancy and sexually transmitted diseases.

Perhaps ironically, inadequate sex education can also create roadblocks to pregnancy. For women, the mystery that surrounds sexuality and reproduction can contribute to infertility in a variety of ways. On the most basic level, if there is ignorance about how conception occurs, it could of course be difficult to get pregnant. More commonly, however, there is a lack of information about how the menstrual cycle works and how it can be thrown off, even among highly educated people. Without this knowledge, many women unknowingly develop conditions that compromise their fertility—conditions that often could be prevented. When they encounter difficulty in getting pregnant, women frequently are directed toward expensive, invasive, and emotionally draining infertility treatments, not realizing that correcting menstrual problems may allow them to get pregnant.

When it comes to taking control of your fertility, education is the first step to empowerment. This chapter will look closely at the female reproductive system and the menstrual cycle, explaining each stage and its role in fertilization. It will also explore the various problems that can interfere with the reproductive process, from hormonal imbalances to thyroid disorders to endometriosis.

You don't have to become a medical expert to enhance your fertility. But understanding the process that leads to conception will help you in pursuing a natural approach to pregnancy.

Getting to Know Your Reproductive Anatomy

It's certainly possible to conceive without knowing much about your reproductive system. But for women who are concerned about their fertility, learning a little about anatomy can go a long way. Here is an overview of your reproductive physiology.

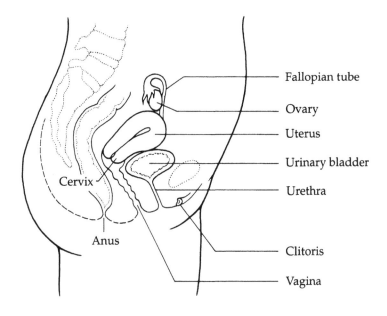

Female reproductive system

Vagina

The vagina is the body's most amazing passageway. It is through the vagina that sperm enter the body during sexual intercourse, menstrual flow leaves the body, and a baby comes into the world. Two sets of lips—known as the labia majora (outer) and the labia minora (inner)—surround the vagina. Above them is the clitoris, the female nerve center for sexual pleasure.

Cervix

Located in the uppermost corner of the vagina, the cervix sits at the entrance to the uterus. It is the reproductive gatekeeper, either ushering in or blocking sperm as they swim in search of a fertile egg. During the menstrual cycle as well as sexual intercourse, the cervix changes position, shape, and texture. It also produces both fertile and infertile mucus at different times during the cycle.

Cervical Os

The cervical os is at the opening of the cervix. Throughout much of the menstrual cycle, the os remains closed. Before ovulation, however, the os opens, then closes once again soon after the egg is released.

Ovaries

About the size of almonds, the ovaries largely control the changes of the menstrual cycle and reproductive hormonal activity in general. These small but powerful glands hold a woman's lifetime supply of eggs, or ova, and also produce the hormones estrogen and progesterone in varying quantities during the menstrual cycle.

Fallopian Tubes

Serving as the passageway for the egg, the fallopian tubes come in a pair, one for each ovary. They constantly sweep back and forth, searching for an egg to transport to the uterus.

Uterus

Commonly known as the womb, the uterus is the fertilized egg's resting place. It is shaped like an upside-down pear, the top of which rests in the vagina. The uterus is the ultimate incubator. It is here that the fertilized egg is deposited by the fallopian tubes. The uterus is where pregnancy begins and where the embryo grows until the time of birth.

Endometrium

The endometrium is the lining of the uterus. After ovulation, the endometrium begins to thicken, preparing for implantation of the fertilized egg. If implantation does not occur, the lining breaks down, resulting in menstruation.

Cervical Mucus

Produced by glands inside the cervix, cervical mucus plays an essential role in reproduction. This fluid can be fertile or non-fertile. Fertile mucus, which is present for several days before ovulation, keeps sperm alive and helps them advance toward the egg. Nonfertile mucus, produced during much of the rest of the menstrual cycle, blocks the passage of sperm.

Menses

The menses is the contents of a woman's menstrual fluid. It is made up of blood, cervical mucus, and the uterine lining, which are all discharged when pregnancy has not occurred.

Corpus Luteum

After ovulation, the sac within the follicle that released the egg transforms into a tiny cyst. This is the corpus luteum, which produces progesterone.

Estrogen

One of the primary reproductive hormones, estrogen is produced by the ovaries and triggers the series of events that lead to ovulation during the first half of the menstrual cycle. The increase of estrogen stimulates egg-containing follicles to develop and tells the cervical glands to secrete fertile mucus. Estrogen is secreted in varying amounts throughout a woman's life.

Progesterone

Also produced by the ovaries, progesterone picks up where estrogen leaves off, increasing after ovulation and prompting the uterine lining to thicken, thus preparing for implantation of the fertilized egg. Like estrogen, it is secreted in varying quantities throughout a woman's life.

Gonadotropin-Releasing Hormone (GnRH)

This hormone is released by the hypothalamus gland in the brain. GnRH gets the ovulatory process going by signaling the pituitary gland to secrete two other hormones: follicle-stimulating hormone and luteinizing hormone.

Follicle-Stimulating Hormone (FSH)

FSH acts on the ovaries, causing a steady flow of estrogen, which in turn leads some of the follicles that hold the eggs to grow and develop. One of these follicles will later release an egg.

Luteinizing Hormone (LH)

Stored by the pituitary gland, LH is the hormone that finally triggers ovulation. A sudden surge of LH floods the ovaries, and within 24 to 36 hours the chosen follicle releases its egg.

How the Menstrual Cycle Works

Every woman has some knowledge about the menstrual cycle. It's part of the feminine birthright, a defining theme of womanhood. By late adolescence, most girls are familiar with the rhythms of their period—when it will come, how heavy the bleeding will be, how long it will last.

Yet the monthly discharge of blood is only the visible evidence of a delicate process that rivals the most advanced human inventions. Repeated hundreds of times over the course of her reproductive life, a woman's menstrual cycle is an amazing example of biological harmony, each element perfectly timed and linked to the greater whole.

The menstrual cycle is divided into two phases. The first, known as the follicular phase, begins with menstruation and continues up to ovulation. The second, called the luteal phase, stretches from ovulation until menstruation. The luteal phase is fixed at 14 days; the follicular phase varies from woman to woman, and sometimes from month to month. During each of the two phases, various changes occur that prepare a woman for the possibility of conception.

The Follicular Phase

This phase takes its name from one of the central players in the menstrual drama—the follicles that house a woman's unfertilized eggs. But let's start at the beginning of the story: menstruation itself.

The monthly cycle opens with the shedding of the previous month's unused reproductive materials, known as the menses. Once the period is over, the hypothalamus—a gland located in the brain—produces gonadotropin-releasing hormone (GnRH). This substance signals the pituitary gland to release follicle-stimulating hormone (FSH). FSH continues the chain reaction, triggering the production of estrogen in the ovaries.

At this point, a number of eggs begin to mature, their growth nurtured by FSH and estrogen. As the levels of estrogen increase, the pituitary releases another hormone. This chemical, called luteinizing hormone (LH), ultimately prompts the follicle containing the chosen egg to release its contents. The result is ovulation, which generally comes 24 to 36 hours after the surge in LH. This is the climax of the menstrual cycle's first phase.

The Luteal Phase

At ovulation, the mature egg begins to make its way to the uterus. This journey is facilitated by the fallopian tubes, the delicate, feathery organs that collect the egg from the ovary. It is in the fallopian tubes that fertilization takes place.

Meanwhile, as soon as ovulation occurs, the shell of the released egg—called the corpus luteum—starts to secrete progesterone. This hormone causes the lining of the uterus, or endometrium, to become rich and thick, preparing it to receive a fertilized egg. Progesterone is also responsible for the rise in basal body temperature, while estrogen alters the fluid known as cervical mucus, making it more hospitable to sperm.

The egg generally lives for up to 24 hours. If fertilization doesn't occur, progesterone production decreases, and the endometrium breaks down. This is the final stage of the menstrual cycle. When the uterine lining starts to flow from the vagina, another cycle has begun.

Cycle Length, Blood Flow, and Irregular Bleeding

The length of the menstrual cycle varies from woman to woman. Some women's cycles are exactly 28 days, but many have shorter or longer cycles. In addition, cycles may change throughout the course of a woman's menstruating years.

Similarly, the amount of flow during menstruation ranges widely, from extremely light to very heavy. A woman's period consists of the discarded uterine lining along with blood and mucus. This explains the often lumpy consistency of the menses.

Some women experience light bleeding between periods. If this happens around ovulation, the cause is often hormonal fluctuation.

There are a number of conditions that may complicate menstruation. Two of the most common are dysmenorrhea, or painful bleeding, and amenorrhea, or the absence of bleeding. Both dysmenorrhea and amenorrhea can be signs of fertility problems.

Many women assume that if they're menstruating, they must be ovulating. But this is not always the case if there is a hormonal imbalance. The menstrual cycle can unfold from start to finish without an egg ever being released. There are several ways to confirm that you are, in fact, ovulating. These

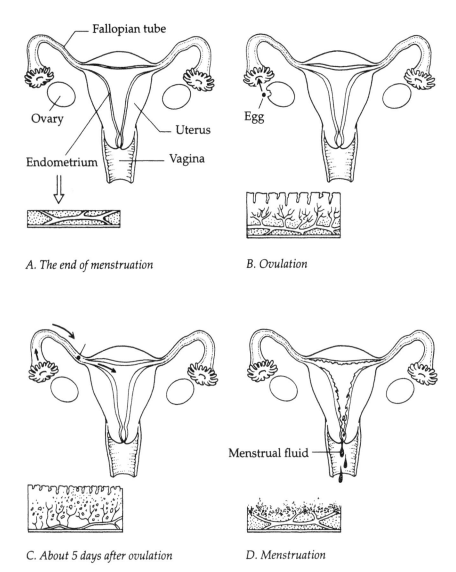

A. *The end of menstruation*

B. *Ovulation*

C. *About 5 days after ovulation*

D. *Menstruation*

The endometrium at four stages in the menstrual cycle

include monitoring basal body temperature, cervical mucus, and LH (see Chapter 5).

It is important to be aware of your menstrual cycle. Healthy women may experience an unusual cycle once or twice a year.

If it happens more frequently, it would be wise to consult a practitioner. Similarly, if you notice abnormal uterine bleeding, unusually long periods of bleeding, or bleeding in between periods, you should see a health care professional. The symptoms may be a direct result of hormonal changes and fluctuations in the body or even structural changes to the uterus and pelvis.

The Male Role in Fertilization

As with women, the reproductive system in men is governed by the pituitary gland. But whereas women are born with a finite number of eggs, men are constantly producing new sperm, which have their own unique life cycle. Here's a summary of the male reproductive process.

The pituitary secretes hormones that signal the testicles to produce sperm and the male hormone testosterone. At puberty a young man will experience beard growth and a lowering of the voice as a result of the body's secretion of testosterone. Interestingly, a man's pituitary will secrete FSH and LH, but not in cycles as with women.

New or immature sperm cells develop in the testicles, then float up into tiny tube-like casings called seminiferous tubules. As they mature, these cells begin to develop a distinct head and tail, resembling a tadpole. The tail is the cell's engine and is designed to propel the sperm through the vagina, cervix, and uterus toward the egg. In a healthy sperm cell the genetic material needed to fertilize an egg is located in the head. The sperm's maturation process takes about 10 weeks.

The sperm leave the testicle when they mature. They must travel through a narrow 12- to 18-foot coiled tube called the epididymis. There are three major glands that contribute fluids that make up semen: the prostate gland, seminal vesicles, and Cowper's glands. Both the semen and the mature sperm empty into a tube called the vas deferens and then into the urethra, which carries the mixture out through the penis during ejaculation. During an average ejaculation a man will expel 150 to 200 million sperm. However, the sperm itself comprise only a very small percentage of the total semen volume, and only about 40 sperm will ever reach the vicinity of an egg.

Chapter 3 will look more closely at factors that can affect male fertility and will discuss the elements of the Six-Step Natural Fertility Program (see Chapter 4) that can benefit men as well as women.

The Journey of the Egg

When a woman's egg and a man's sperm successfully merge, the end result is truly miraculous. Yet because we don't generally examine this miracle when it happens, we tend to take the complicated nature of conception for granted.

Indeed, it's no simple task to conceive. Once the egg has been released into the fallopian tubes, there's a brief window of fertility. During the next 12 to 24 hours, a sperm must overcome numerous obstacles and penetrate the membrane containing the mature egg.

Once successfully fertilized, the egg resumes its journey to the uterus. By the time it arrives, the endometrium should be rich enough in progesterone for implantation to take place. If it isn't, the embryo will not be able to implant itself, and the fertilized egg will be lost. Here are the various stages of the egg's journey, from ovulation to fertilization to implantation.

Stage 1 The process begins when the pituitary gland releases two hormones: follicle-stimulating hormone (FSH) and luteinizing hormone (LH). The release of these two hormones signals the ovary to start developing and maturing an egg.

Stage 2   Ovulation is the next step in the process. An elevated estrogen level and a surge in LH prompt the follicle to open and release the mature egg.

Stage 3   The egg now moves from the ovary into the fallopian tube. Feathery organs known as fimbria reach down and draw the egg into the tube.

Stage 4   The egg is fertilized by the sperm. The result is called the zygote.

Stage 5   The zygote, containing chromosomes from both mother and father, divides. The zygote is becoming an embryo.

Stage 6   More natural fluids are released into the fallopian tube, assisting fertilization and cell division. The embryo continues its journey down the fallopian tube.

Stage 7   The embryo arrives in the uterus and implants itself into the uterine wall, where it will continue to grow.

Hormones—A Delicate Balance

Hormones are the chemicals that regulate most of the body's internal functions, including body temperature, digestion, sexual development, and reproduction. The functions related to reproduction are controlled by the reproductive endocrine system, a collection of glands that produce hormones. These hormones are secreted into the bloodstream, which carries them to their respective destinations throughout the body. The endocrine system is so complex that some hormones serve only to stimulate certain glands, which in turn produce other hormones.

The two primary female hormones are estrogen and progesterone, both of which are produced by the ovaries. At puberty, the body's estrogen levels increase to enhance secondary sex characteristics, such as breast growth and widening hips. Estrogen also stimulates the hypothalamus gland, which is located at the base of the brain. This is where the body produces gonadotropin-releasing hormone (GnRH). The secretion of GnRH begins the process of ovulation.

All of the key reproductive hormones—estrogen, progesterone, GnRH, FSH, and LH—must be in sync with one another. If the balance is thrown off even slightly, ovulation can be affected. Much of the focus of infertility treatment is on restoring hormonal balance.

What Can Go Wrong

Reproduction is a complex symphony of male and female biology. A woman's endocrine system must be performing normally, secreting the exact level of hormones at the exact times on a regular, cyclical basis. The ovaries must be able to produce at least one mature egg follicle each month. They must release the egg at the proper juncture in the menstrual cycle. This egg must contain the right amount of genetic material for successful fertilization. The fallopian tubes must be free and clear of obstructions and must be able to catch and propel the egg toward the uterus.

Likewise, a man's sperm has to contain many healthy, strong-swimming sperm. Even the semen must be able to transform from a jelly-like substance to a liquid 30 to 40 minutes after ejaculation. The sperm must be introduced into a woman's reproductive system around ovulation, a window of opportunity that ranges from 3 to 5 days each month.

In addition, the cervix must produce enough fertile mucus to protect, nourish, and transport sperm toward the uterine chamber and up into the fallopian tubes. The uterus must be unobstructed and free of scar tissue or lesions, its walls thick and healthy enough to allow the fertilized egg to embed itself and grow. After conception and implantation, the hormonal system must continue to work smoothly, creating a secure environment for the placenta to develop and nourish the growing fetus.

Even the slightest disturbance in this intricate system can thwart conception. So it's easy to see why a fertile couple has only a 20% chance of conceiving per cycle, and more than one-third of pregnancies are lost spontaneously, often before the woman even realizes she's pregnant. But with regular inter-course, as many as 80% of fertile couples will become pregnant within 12 months.

THE SIX BASIC BIOLOGICAL FUNCTIONS THAT MUST BE PRESENT FOR CONCEPTION TO OCCUR

- Healthy pelvis and pelvic organs
- Normal cervical function
- Normal uterine function
- Normal fallopian tube function
- Regular ovulation
- Good sperm count and motility

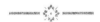

What Can Go Wrong in Women

Here are some of the reproductive conditions that can inter-fere with a woman's fertility.

Endometriosis

One of the most common causes of female infertility is endometriosis, which afflicts an estimated 5 to 10 million women in the United States alone (about 7% of the overall female population). Endometriosis is a chronic, often painful, and unpredictable condition. It has been reported in 25% to 50% of infertile women.

Endometriosis does not always pose a problem for conception. In fact, some women have had one or more children only to find out later that they had asymptomatic endometriosis. However, for others it can be the key factor in preventing pregnancy.

Endometriosis occurs when pieces of the endometrium or uterine lining migrate or grow outside the uterus. These pieces then attach themselves to the ovaries, the fallopian tubes, or other parts of the pelvic cavity. Symptoms range from severe menstrual cramping to pain during intercourse. The primary symptom of endometriosis is dysmenorrhea, accompanied by dull, aching pain in the pelvis, lower abdomen, and back.

"Once the endometrial cells are transplanted, they still respond to the monthly hormonal messages just as they would if remaining in the uterus—by filling with blood, which is then released at the time of menses," says John Lee, M.D., of Sebastopol, California. "The drops of blood, however, have nowhere to go and can become a focus of excruciating pain and inflammation. Despite their small size—some are no larger than a pinhead—the pelvic pain that results can be disabling. Symptoms tend to increase gradually over the years as the endometriosis areas slowly increase in size."

Current thinking on the cause of endometriosis is that it may be one of many autoimmune diseases that affect women. According to Carolyn DeMarco, M.D., of Toronto, Canada, this means that the body is rejecting the abnormal endometrial tissue in the pelvis and giving off both localized and general symptoms. Recent studies have shown that the immune system of women with endometriosis is depressed.

Christiane Northrup, M.D., of Yarmouth, Maine, notes that every woman probably has embryonic cells that could potentially develop into endometrial tissue. This view is shared by David Redwine, M.D., of Bend, Oregon, a gynecologist who has conducted extensive research on the causes and treatments of endometriosis. Dr. Redwine's theory is that endometriosis is a static condition that women are born with as a result of cell buildup on the uterine wall, possibly left behind during fetal development. As a woman enters reproductive maturity, certain factors result in the disease becoming active.

Dr. DeMarco believes that environmental contaminants such as dioxin, radiation, and other industrial chemicals top the list of culprits. Other factors, she says, include stress; a diet high in animal fat; deficiencies in iodine, essential fatty acids, and certain vitamins and minerals; candidiasis; poor liver function; and progesterone shortages.

According to Dr. DeMarco, endometriosis is also linked to hereditary factors. "Endometriosis is carried on the mother's side, and a [woman with a] first-degree relative with endometriosis has a three to twelve times greater chance of having endometriosis."

For most women, the symptom that brings them into the doctor's office is pelvic pain. The pain, however, is not localized. Some women in Dr. Redwine's study had painful periods, while others reported pain during sex, bowel movements, aerobic exercise, and posture changes. One-fifth reported no symptoms at all.

Despite its prevalence and often debilitating effects, endometriosis often goes untreated by doctors. According to Dr. Redwine, over three-fourths of the women he has treated for endometriosis had been dismissed by their primary physicians as being neurotic.

The first step in diagnosing endometriosis is a thorough pelvic examination. If the condition is present, the ligaments supporting the uterus are often tender and sometimes have developed small lumps. A definitive diagnosis can be made with a biopsy of the endometrial tissue. Dr. DeMarco adds that an ultrasound may also provide evidence of the disease.

Treatment options span the full range of medical care, from prescriptive hormone manipulation to various alternative therapies to surgical procedures.

Hormonal Imbalance

At least 25% of infertile women suffer from some sort of hormonal imbalance and dysfunction. If the pituitary produces insufficient levels of follicle-stimulating hormone (FSH), a woman will not produce an egg follicle. If there is no surge of luteinizing hormone (LH), the egg will not be released.

If these imbalances happen sporadically, the condition is called ovulatory dysfunction. It is far more common than involution, a condition where a woman never ovulates. The system is so sensitive that even when ovulation occurs, if there is insufficient progesterone from the corpus luteum, a message will be sent indicating that the endometrium is incapable of sustaining a fertilized egg. This is known as a luteal phase defect.

The reasons behind hormonal imbalance are not always clear. Thyroid disease, poor nutrition and eating disorders such as anorexia nervosa and bulimia, stress, and polycystic ovarian disease are some of the possible causes. Although hormonal therapies are quite effective, alternative approaches such as acupuncture, herbal remedies, and homeopathy can be equally successful and put less strain on the body, as we'll discuss in later chapters.

Pelvic Inflammatory Disease (PID)

A major factor in fertility problems is pelvic inflammatory disease, or PID. Caused most frequently by sexually transmitted diseases, PID can affect the cervix, the fallopian tubes, the ovaries, and the uterus.

PID infects and inflames a woman's reproductive system.

Often hard to diagnose in the early stages, it is probably most frequently detected in an asymptomatic stage during routine examinations. When the disease becomes active, its most common symptom is lower abdominal pain.

Chlamydia and gonorrhea are the leading causes of PID. Though these conditions can be treated effectively, both are often asymptomatic and therefore go undetected. Other causes include the use of an intrauterine device (IUD), douching, surgical procedures such as abortion, and childbirth. Smoking has also been linked to a higher incidence of PID.

If PID reaches the fallopian tubes, it can result in blockage of the tubes, thus preventing pregnancy. Another danger associated with PID is ectopic pregnancy, where the embryo is implanted in the fallopian tubes. This can lead to a life-threatening rupture.

If caught early, PID responds to noninvasive treatment with one or more prescription antibiotics. In some cases, however, surgery is required to repair damage done to reproductive organs. As with many conditions that affect fertility, prevention is the key with PID. Using barrier contraceptive devices such as condoms and diaphragms is the most effective way of avoiding PID. Regular gynecological examinations are also important as a means of early detection.

Ovarian Cysts and Polycystic Ovarian Disease (PCOD)

If a woman isn't ovulating, cysts form in the ovaries. This condition is known as polycystic ovarian disease (PCOD).

PCOD is strongly associated with obesity and an excess of the hormone androgen. While androgen occurs naturally in women, an overabundance creates confusion within the endocrine system, ultimately preventing release of the egg from the ovaries and causing secondary symptoms such as weight gain and abnormal hair growth. Eventually, the ovaries become filled with cysts formed by the follicles that contained the immature eggs.

PCOD can be treated with prescription medications or a combination of dietary changes, nutritional supplementation, alternative therapies, and/or exercise. In severe cases, surgery may be necessary.

Luteal-Phase Problems

This condition refers to the second phase of the menstrual cycle following ovulation, when the uterus is preparing for possible implantation of a fertilized egg. If the endometrial lining does not develop properly, implantation is impossible. Luteal-phase problems result from hormonal imbalances or irregularities in the endometrium. They can be treated with a range of alternative and conventional therapies.

Obstruction of the Fallopian Tubes

Problems in the fallopian tubes are generally the result of infections associated with either sexually transmitted diseases or intrauterine devices (IUDs). Infection can lead to structural damage of the tubes, interfering with ovulation. Medication can treat this condition, but it must be caught early.

Ovarian Failure

A relatively small number of infertility cases can be traced directly to a problem in the ovaries. Congenital defects can render the ovaries unable to function properly, as can autoimmune conditions and pelvic infections. Whereas infections can be treated with medication, there is no effective treatment for congenital and autoimmune ovarian problems.

Abortion

Dilatation and curettage (D&C), the procedure used in the majority of abortions, can cause damage to the cervix that may lead to fertility problems. In some cases, scar tissue that forms after the surgery results in a narrowing of the cervical opening; the glands that produce cervical mucus may also be affected by scar tissue developed following an abortion. Either of these conditions can make it difficult for sperm to pass through the cervix and into the uterus. Treatment depends on the extent of the damage and may involve both alternative and conventional techniques.

Diethylstilbestrol (DES)

The drug DES was commonly used in the 1950s to prevent miscarriages. Only later was it discovered that DES was responsible for a number of serious health problems. Among them is infertility in the children of mothers who used the medication. DES infertility is typically associated with abnormalities in the reproductive organs, including the uterus, cervix, and fallopian tubes. The severity of the problem and whether it will respond to treatment depends on the DES dosage that was taken and for how long, as well as when the drug was taken during the pregnancy.

Cervical Mucus Problems

Just before and during ovulation, a woman's cervical mucus plays a key role in the fertilization process, providing a welcoming environment for the advancing sperm. If no fertile mucus is being produced, sperm will not be able to advance into the uterus and fallopian tubes. This problem is diagnosed with an examination of the cervical mucus, performed by a practitioner after the woman has had intercourse. A range of alternative and conventional therapies are available.

Other Cervical Problems

Many doctors perform surgical procedures upon finding abnormalities during a Pap smear. These procedures are often not necessary and can cause damage to the cervix, which may lead to infertility. Problematic Pap smears can frequently be treated with medication, thereby avoiding the risks of surgery; if the condition persists, less traumatic procedures are available that will also reduce the chance of cervical damage.

Sexually Transmitted Diseases (STDs)

STDs are at epidemic proportions and are a major cause of fertility problems. Conditions range from HIV/AIDS (human immunodeficiency virus/acquired immunodeficiency syndrome), syphilis, and gonorrhea to herpes, genital warts, and chlamydia. If left untreated, these infections can cause major reproductive damage. Although prevention is the best approach, most STDs can be effectively controlled with medication when caught early.

Vaginitis

Yeast infections, along with conditions such as trichomoniasis and *Gardnerella*, can also lead to infertility. The various forms of vaginitis affect a woman's vaginal health, making it more difficult for sperm to reach the egg. They can be effectively treated with alternative and conventional therapies.

Ectopic Pregnancy

An ectopic pregnancy occurs when the fertilized egg develops in the fallopian tubes rather than the uterus. This is a potentially life-threatening condition and must be treated as quickly as possible, either with medication or surgery. Ectopic pregnancies affect only a small percentage of women, although those who have had tubal or pelvic surgery or tubal damage are at higher risk. Since an ectopic pregnancy may harm the fallopian tube, subsequent pregnancy may be more difficult to achieve.

The Uterus Factor

Even when a woman's ovaries and fallopian tubes are in good working order, pregnancy may still be prevented by uterine problems. These include uterine cysts, fibroids, and adhesions, any of which can interfere with implantation of the embryo. If implantation occurs, uterine difficulties remain a potential obstacle. In some cases, the cervix can't support the weight of an embryo. In others, intrauterine infections lead to miscarriages. Uterine problems can be treated with a variety of alternative and conventional therapies, depending on the specific condition.

Immunological Infertility

Most sperm never make it close to the unfertilized egg, succumbing to a woman's natural defenses. In some cases of infertility, however, all of the sperm become inactive while still in the vagina because of a condition known as immunological infertility. This occurs when no distinction is made between sperm, on the one hand, and viruses or bacteria, on the other. Thus, the sperm are targeted for destruction by a woman's immune system, preventing pregnancy.

Birth-Control Pills

These contraceptive agents prevent pregnancy by altering a woman's hormonal function. Even after she stops using the pill, a woman may continue to experience hormonal irregularities that can interfere with menstruation and ovulation. In addition, the pill can lead to nutrient deficiencies that also can cause menstrual and ovulatory problems. For this reason, a postpill supplement regime (discussed in Chapter 6) is advisable to help restore proper menstrual function.

Douching

Douching can have a negative impact on fertility in several ways. Women who douche right before intercourse may make the vagina either too acidic or too alkaline, while those who douche immediately following sex run the risk of rinsing out their partner's sperm. Douching around the time of menstruation has also been linked to a higher incidence of PID. However, women whose vaginal pH levels are too high or too low may benefit from natural douches, according to Niels H. Lauersen, M.D.

Menstrual Health—The Key to Conception

There are women who go through their lives without any menstrual troubles. At some point, however, most women experience menstrual difficulties of one kind or another. In many cases, the problem is minor and will not lead to further health problems. In other situations, menstrual conditions— even ones that may seem mild—can pose an obstacle to pregnancy.

Maintaining optimal menstrual and reproductive health is the best way to enhance your fertility. Chapter 4 will introduce you to the six-step fertility program, which can help you treat menstrual problems or even prevent them. By using the combination of alternative therapies described in our program, most women can increase their menstrual well-being and improve their chances of healthy conception.

CHAPTER THREE

Male Fertility

Compared to the complex nature of female fertility, the male role in reproduction might seem rather straightforward. On one level, this is true: if a man is producing strong, healthy sperm in normal quantities, he is generally fertile.

But that's a big "if." In some 40% of infertility cases, the problem can be traced to the man. And in another 20%, either a combination of male and female factors or unexplained causes are responsible.

At first, the idea that he is not fertile may be difficult for a man to grasp. Whereas women often have clear symptoms related to infertility, men may not. So it's natural for them to assume that if they can ejaculate, they can also procreate.

Of course, the presence of semen is no assurance of fertility. The only way to determine male fertility is through laboratory tests that measure not only sperm quantity but also motility, or the speed at which sperm swim. Semen analysis also reveals whether sperm may have some structural irregularity that is interfering with conception.

Just as women's reproductive function is dependent on a host of factors, multiple elements influence sperm health. In this chapter, we'll look at the various conditions that can compromise male fertility, what causes them, and how they can be treated with many aspects of the Six-Step Natural Fertility Program.

Conditions That Cause Male Infertility

Varicoceles

A varicocele is a varicose vein in a testicle. This condition can lead to increased temperature in the scrotum, which in turn can decrease sperm production. A varicocele is easily detected by an examination of the testicles and can be corrected with minor surgery.

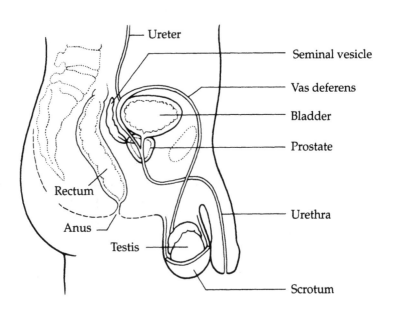

Male reproductive organs

Hypospadia

Hypospadia is a congenital condition in which the urethra opening is on the underside of the penis. As a result, when the man ejaculates during intercourse, the semen is released lower in the vagina, decreasing the chances that his sperm will make it into the uterus. Hypospadia can generally be repaired through surgery.

Cryptorchidism

A small percentage of boys are born with cryptorchidism, or undescended testicles. Once again, surgery is required to correct the problem.

Klinefelter's Syndrome

Klinefelter's syndrome is a genetic defect in which a man carries an extra X chromosome, causing sterility. No treatment is available.

Congenital Absence of Vas Deferens

The vas deferens is the duct through which semen is ejaculated. If a man is born without it, he cannot impregnate a woman through intercourse. However, since he still produces semen, sperm can be collected from the epididymis, which stores sperm, and used for in vitro fertilization.

The Mumps

This common childhood ailment can cause infertility in adult men by crippling sperm production. Those at risk include men who have never had the mumps or who were not vaccinated against the disease.

Other Infections

Viral and bacterial infections such as prostatitis, urethritis, epididymitis, gonorrhea, and chlamydia can also lead to infertility and should be treated promptly.

Sports Injuries

The male reproductive anatomy is vulnerable to a variety of athletic accidents. According to Niels H. Lauersen, M.D., these include a ruptured epididymis, split or torn vas deferens, shattered testicles, injured seminal vesicles and/or prostate gland, bladder damage, and back trauma that restricts sexual activity.

Hormonal Problems

Although often overlooked, male hormonal imbalance can lead to fertility problems. A shortage of testosterone is one potential roadblock. In rarer cases, insufficient follicle-stimulating hormone (FSH) and luteinizing hormone (LH) can prevent the production of sperm.

Sperm Duct Blockage

A man can ejaculate into a woman, but if the semen doesn't contain any sperm, it won't do much good. A sperm duct blockage can create just such a scenario by preventing the sperm from getting to the urethra. Surgery can sometimes correct the problem.

Antisperm Antibodies

Women are not the only ones who can wipe out sperm with antibodies. In some cases, men develop antibodies that target their own sperm.

Retrograde Ejaculation

This condition occurs when sperm travels backward rather than forward, depositing itself in a man's bladder. For obvious reasons, retrograde ejaculation makes conception impossible.

Sexual Dysfunction

Getting and maintaining an erection is a prerequisite for ejaculation. If a man suffers from periodic or chronic impotence, his fertility will be compromised.

Unexplained Infertility

As with women, men can be infertile with no known explanation. In fact, according to Richard Marrs, M.D., the majority of male infertility cases fall into this category. Although unexplained infertility is harder to treat, it does not mean a man is unable to impregnate his partner.

Factors That Influence Male Fertility

Male fertility can be affected by a wide range of factors. Here are the most common problems.

Drugs

Recreational drugs such as marijuana, cocaine, and heroin pose one of the greatest threats to sperm health. In fact, this is the major factor queried in all fertility workups. Street drugs, in particular, are harmful to male fertility. Many prescription drugs, including antidepressants and blood-pressure medications, can also have detrimental effects on sperm formation, as can anabolic steroids.

Smoking

Another major risk factor for male fertility is smoking. Even if the man hasn't been smoking for years, there may be long-lasting damage to sperm.

Alcohol

Not only does alcohol decrease testosterone and promote the conversion of testosterone to estrogen, but excessive long-term use can create varicoceles—one of the leading causes of male infertility.

Stress

Stress, anxiety, and depression can all interfere with hormonal function, thus affecting sperm formation. Testicular and prostate health are both negatively impacted by stress, which damages cell growth and thus sperm development.

Excessive Ejaculation

Sperm counts can be depleted by too-frequent masturbation or intercourse. What constitutes ejaculatory excess depends largely on the man's constitution. Some people are fine if they masturbate or have intercourse every day, whereas some would have a problem if they ejaculated once a week. If a low sperm count is found, it's important for the man to be honest with his practitioner about his sexual habits. Otherwise, a couple may waste a lot of time, energy, and money trying to diagnose and treat infertility that's easily resolved through lifestyle change.

Heat

Prolonged exposure to elevated temperatures is one of the greatest risk factors for male fertility. In order to produce healthy sperm, the testicles need to be remain cooler than the rest of the body, which is why they hang down. Among the activities to be avoided are excessive hot tub use and riding a motorcycle. Tight-fitting clothes, particularly underwear, may also generate too much heat for optimum testes health.

Weight

Obesity can impair sperm production by interfering with normal hormonal function as well as creating too much vascular burden, leading to varicoceles.

Excessive or Inadequate Exercise

By contributing to healthy circulation and endocrine function, exercise can help protect fertility. Extreme fitness routines, however, can have the opposite effect, straining the glandular system and depriving the body of adequate nutrition for healthy sperm production.

Poor Diet

Men with poor eating habits may not have the nutrients necessary for healthy reproductive function. Vitamins A, B, C, and E are all essential for male fertility, as are the minerals zinc, selenium, and chromium. Essential fatty acids also play a vital role, along with amino acids.

Caffeine

Although studies have been inconclusive, many doctors believe that, based on clinical experience, excessive caffeine intake can be a factor in male fertility problems.

Environmental Toxins

A growing body of research indicates that men exposed to various workplace hazards, including certain pesticides and industrial chemicals, may be at risk for infertility.

BIKING, UNDERWEAR, AND INFERTILITY

The medical community is split on whether heavy bicycle riding can lower a man's sperm count. But a conservative approach probably is the best course. Excessive bicycle riding creates prostate irritation, but it is not yet known if it also creates testicular irritation. In addition to cutting down on riding, buying a seat that minimizes pressure on the groin is suggested.

Tight-fitting briefs are also thought by many to put a damper on male fertility. No clear consensus exists on whether underwear affects sperm production, but many practitioners advise their male patients to hang loose. Tight underwear is thought to create undue heat retention.

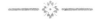

Maintaining and Restoring Male Fertility

Good overall health is the best place to start with female fertility, and the same holds true for men. "I try to get the person generally healthy and then deal with the reproductive issues," says Roger Hirsh, O.M.D., L.Ac., of Beverly Hills, California. "If you get them healthy, you're addressing the endocrine and adrenal systems anyway."

"In Chinese medicine, we view symptoms associated with male fertility problems as fatigue, erectile difficulties, decreased sexual desire, coldness or pain in the lower back, weak knees, and frequent nighttime urination." To get an accurate picture of what's going on, the first step is a semen analysis. Dr. Hirsh considers normal sperm volume to be 50 million per cubic centimeter, and normal motility to be 60% to 80%.

Once low count, poor motility, and/or other sperm irregularities are detected, a variety of alternative therapies are available that can help restore a man's fertility. Here are some of the many options.

Diet and Nutritional Supplementation

It's important for men to consume a healthy diet, especially if they are experiencing fertility problems. Indeed, medical studies have found a strong relationship between nutrition and sperm health.

The general principles of a whole-foods diet (explained in Chapter 6) apply to both genders. However, men and women do have somewhat different needs when it comes to fertility. In their excellent book *Encyclopedia of Natural Medicine*, Michael Murray, N.D., and Joseph Pizzorno, N.D., offer the following dietary guidelines for male infertility:

- Avoid saturated fats, hydrogenated oils, transfatty acids, and cottonseed oil, all of which can lead to free radical damage.
- Increase intake of legumes (especially soy products), foods high in antioxidants, carotenes and flavonoids (dark-colored vegetables and fruits), and essential fatty acids.
- Eat 8 to 10 servings of vegetables, 2 to 4 servings of fresh fruit, and one-half cup of raw nuts or seeds daily.

Dr. Murray and Dr. Pizzorno also recommend daily supplements for male infertility:

High-potency multiple vitamin-and-mineral supplement

Vitamin C: 500–3000 milligrams (three times per day)

Vitamin E: 600–800 international units

Beta-carotene: 100,000 to 200,000 international units

Folic Acid: 400 micrograms

Vitamin B_{12}: 1000 micrograms

Zinc: 30–60 milligrams

The amino acids arginine and lysine are both associated with male reproductive health. Supplements of 500 milligrams a day may help improve fertility.

SUPPLEMENTING FOR SEXUAL VITALITY

Fertility and sexual drive are closely related, so it's not surprising that certain nutrients are essential to maintain sexual vitality. In her book *Love Potions*, Cynthia M. Watson, M.D., recommends the following supplements for men:

Vitamin B_1: 50–100 milligrams

Vitamin B_2: 50–100 milligrams

Vitamin B_3: 50–500 milligrams

Vitamin B_5: 50–1000 milligrams

Vitamin B_6: 50–100 milligrams

Vitamin B_{12}: 100 micrograms

Folic Acid: 800 micrograms

Choline: 500–3000 milligrams

Vitamin C: 1000–5000 milligrams

Bioflavonoids: 200–1000 milligrams

Vitamin A: 5000–10,000 international units

Beta-carotene: 15,000–25,000 international units

Vitamin E: 400–800 international units

Calcium: 500–1000 milligrams

Magnesium: 500 milligrams

Zinc: 30–100 milligrams

Selenium: 100–200 micrograms

Chromium: 200–500 micrograms

Iodine: 150 micrograms

Manganese: 10 milligrams

Phenylalanine: 500–3000 milligrams

Arginine: 100–6000 milligrams

Herbal Medicine

Herbs have long been used in the treatment of both male and female infertility. Here are some of the more common ones for men. Consult with a practitioner to determine dosages and the best form for each.

Panax Ginseng This popular herb is known to promote hormonal activity, including testosterone, and is generally regarded as a powerful chi, or energy, tonic, according to Jill Stansbury, N.D., of Battle Ground, Washington. She notes that studies have shown ginseng to increase sperm count.

Ashwagandha Also known as Indian ginseng, ashwagandha has similar properties to Chinese ginseng.

Saw Palmetto This well-known herb can be effective in cases of infertility linked to conditions of the prostate gland, including prostatic hypertrophy and prostatitis. It can also be helpful for erectile dysfunction and is a good tonic for the reproductive organs and the urinary tract.

Pygeum Like saw palmetto, pygeum may improve fertility in cases where the prostate is affected.

Ginkgo Infertility stemming from circulatory problems may benefit from ginkgo, since blood flow difficulties can lead to erectile dysfunction.

Hawthorn Another circulatory tonic as well as an antioxidant, hawthorn may be useful for men with blood vessel disease or hypertension.

Sarsaparilla This herb is thought to be androgen-promoting, heightening adrenal gland function and raising testosterone levels. Dr. Stansbury notes that sarsaparilla is a blood-cleansing herb that promotes liver detoxification and thus may boost reproductive function, since the liver metabolizes hormones and helps control their levels.

Garlic The antioxidant properties of garlic may favor fertility by protecting sperm from free radical damage. Garlic can also be useful for impotence.

Licorice This herb works as a tonic for the adrenal glands and reproductive organs and can stimulate hormonal activity.

Damiana Damiana is used primarily to spur sexual desire in both men and women.

False Unicorn Root This general reproductive tonic can help correct impotence.

Chinese Herbs In traditional Chinese medicine, herbs are a key part of treatment for male infertility. By improving circulation and strengthening the liver, herbal remedies help increase sperm count, motility, and health. Generally, several herbs are combined into a formula. Consult with an herbalist or doctor of Oriental medicine to obtain the appropriate formula for your condition.

Chapter 7 offers more general information about herbal medicine.

Aromatherapy

In her book *Enhancing Fertility Naturally*, health writer and childbirth educator Nicki Wesson recommends the following aromatherapy oils for male infertility:

Thyme

Cumin

Basil

Cedarwood

Vetiver

Angelica

Sage

Clary Sage

Bergamot

Black Pepper

Geranium

Aromatherapy is discussed in more detail in Chapter 7.

Acupuncture

Acupuncture is an integral part of the traditional Chinese medicine approach to male fertility issues. "Most treatments for male infertility address the kidney system," explains Daoshing Ni, O.M.D., L.Ac., of Santa Monica, California. "In

Chinese medicine, the kidney system translates into the reproductive system."

In addition to enhancing kidney function, acupuncture treatments also help stimulate the liver and activate blood circulation. Points may be in the lower back, the lower legs, the pelvis, or other areas, depending on the patient and the specific problem.

Acupuncture is reviewed fully in Chapter 7.

Homeopathy

In her book *Getting Pregnant Naturally*, health writer Winifred Conkling offers a useful overview of homeopathic remedies for both male and female infertility. Common remedies for men include the following:

Agnus For erectile difficulties or lack of energy.

Conium For erectile difficulties accompanied by cramping and coldness in the legs.

Graphites For loss of sexual desire or ejaculatory problems.

Lycopodium For insecurity and performance anxiety that interfere with strong sexual desire.

Nitric acidium For loss of sexual desire accompanied by irritability, self-criticism, and sensitivity to criticism.

Nux vomica For ejaculatory problems possibly accompanied by a short temper and impatience.

Phosphoric acidium For loss of sexual desire.

Sepia For loss of sexual desire accompanied by a dragging sensation in the genitals.

Homeopathy is discussed in more detail in Chapter 7.

Exercise

Physical activity is an important part of general health. It can also contribute to optimal male fertility by maintaining strong circulation and endocrine function.

While most kinds of exercise are beneficial, fitness routines that both strengthen and relax the body can be particularly helpful for men facing fertility problems. Yoga, chi gung, and tai chi—discussed in Chapter 8—all fall into this category.

In chi gung, the key to male fertility is energy. "Chi gung is about gathering energy, conserving energy, and transforming energy," explains Roger Jahnke, O.M.D., L.Ac., of Santa Barbara, California. "In the male context, all three of these are very primary."

According to Dr. Jahnke, chi gung practice can help restore depleted adrenal glands. When the adrenals are overly taxed, reproductive function suffers. "Daily practice is going to be a positive component of the recovery from any kind of sexual challenge," he says. Male fertility problems can result from a variety of pathogenic factors, including stress, emotional upset, overexertion, and excessive sexual activity. Chi gung aids the body in recovering from these imbalances.

Specific exercises for male fertility focus on a group of muscles inside the pelvis at the top of the leg. By contracting these muscles, both sexual and reproductive function can be enhanced.

Massage is another powerful stress-reduction technique with implications for both male and female infertility (see Chapter 8). Dr. Ni recommends self-massage of the testicles to improve circulation, which can stimulate sperm production.

Conserving Male Sexual Energy

Jing is the Chinese word for male resources, including hormones, DNA (deoxyribonucleic acid), ATP (adenosine triphosphate), and semen. "The Chinese feel that the human system has a certain amount of jing available to be spent," says Dr. Jahnke. "When we spend in the sexual act, we're basically depleting the jing pool."

For young, healthy men under 25, depleting the jing supply is generally not a concern. As men get older, however, excessive ejaculation can lead to a jing deficit. "The same sexual habits over 25 become a problem. That tangles in with overworking, even overplaying, and then becomes a very strong cause for imbalance in the system, particularly in the hormonal system, including low sperm, bad motility, low libido."

For men, part of chi gung practice is conserving their sexual energy by sometimes refraining from ejaculation. In combination with a good diet, adequate rest, and overall healthy lifestyle, this approach can maintain male sexual vigor. "The rule is to have a high level of vitality in your life, and then on those occasions when you do ejaculate to have a quick recovery to a high level of vitality," explains Dr. Jahnke. In cases where men are already experiencing symptoms such as low libido or low sperm count and motility, he also recommends acupuncture and herbs to help restore sexual health.

Mind/Body Medicine

Men can benefit from the stress-reduction techniques of mind/body medicine discussed in detail in Chapter 9.

A Man's Role

As we've seen, male factors play a major part in whether conception can occur, which is sufficient reason for men to be closely involved in maintaining or restoring fertility. It's equally important on an emotional level for men to be active in the quest for pregnancy. Couples who pursue this journey together not only stand a better chance of achieving the goal of pregnancy but will preserve and strengthen their relationship.

CHAPTER FOUR

The Six-Step Natural Fertility Program

Now that you have a better understanding of what infertility means and what can cause it, you're almost ready to begin the program. Below you'll read a description of the six steps recommended for a natural approach to fertility. By following this plan, you will:

- Improve your overall feelings of health and well-being
- Learn to prevent, control, or reverse conditions that can impair fertility
- Reduce stress and anxiety
- Create balance in your life
- Prepare your body, mind, and spirit for pregnancy

Before getting started, there are a few very important issues to consider. Thinking carefully about these matters will have a significant influence on the effectiveness of the program.

Making the Time, Making the Commitment

In today's world, most women lead very busy lives. Between work, friends, and family responsibilities, it may feel as if there's little time for anything else. If busy describes your life, you may need to make an attitude shift before doing anything else. Think of it as giving yourself the time of your life.

For this program to truly serve you, you will need to make time to take care of yourself. A natural approach to fertility isn't just another thing to squeeze into a hectic schedule. It may require some fundamental lifestyle changes—better eating, regular exercise, relaxation, adequate sleep—for which there are no shortcuts.

This doesn't mean that you have to drop everything in order to get pregnant. But you may need to reexamine your priorities and cut back in some areas so that you have enough time to devote to your physical and emotional health.

Initially, these changes might seem challenging, even unwelcome. But you'll quickly come to appreciate how valuable it is to clear time and space for yourself, and you'll realize how good it feels to lead a more balanced life.

Hand in hand with making time for the program is making the commitment. This is not a commitment to some abstract routine—it is a commitment to yourself.

Despite the social advances of the past few decades, women are still taught to be caretakers. Too often this translates into focusing on others at the expense of themselves. Sure, women are free to pursue careers today in a way that their mothers and grandmothers were not. But they still tend to get stuck with a disproportionate amount of housework, as well as being counted upon to fulfill time-consuming obligations to friends and family. The result for many is a hectic lifestyle in which their own needs always seem to come last.

The Six-Step Natural Fertility Program proposes a different approach. To prepare your body, mind, and spirit for pregnancy, you can begin with nurturing yourself. You must not only make the time but affirm the necessity of attending to your needs.

Following the program will probably require that you do a little less for others than you're accustomed to, and that you ask for a little more in return. Cutting back a bit on work is a good place to start. Giving yourself a few extra hours a week can make a big difference, whether that time is spent exercising, reading, cooking an enjoyable meal, or simply relaxing.

Again, it might be hard at first, but you'll soon realize that acknowledging and accommodating your needs is neither selfish nor indulgent. On the contrary, as your health and vitality improve, so too will your ability to take care of those you love.

Working with the Program

The goal of the Six-Step Natural Fertility Program is to help you get pregnant naturally. But it is also designed to give you a greater sense of overall well-being. The last thing you need is a long list of new "to do's," and the steps outlined in the following chapters need not be viewed in this way. They are meant to provide you with the knowledge and options to enable you to take control of your own fertility. Each step can be adapted to your own specific feelings and circumstances.

Keep in mind that these guidelines should be used in consultation with your physician or health care practitioner. They are not intended to take the place of professional care.

How to Choose a Doctor or Health Care Practitioner

Selecting a doctor or other health care professional who will work with you is a vital part of the program. Establishing this relationship before starting will help you get the best results.

Building a strong partnership with a practitioner can play a major role in your overall health and in your efforts to get pregnant naturally. In addition to providing care and information, the medical professional you choose will ideally be a source of support who will help guide you through sometimes complex decisions. For this reason, compatibility between patient and practitioner can be a major factor in the healing process.

Before looking for the right match, however, it's essential to understand your own role in improving your health. Although finding a good doctor is important, the truth is that you hold the keys to your physical and emotional well-being. This may sound intimidating at first, but taking responsibility for your body can be immensely empowering. By asserting control over your health care, the feeling of helplessness that so many people experience when dealing with medical issues will be replaced by a sense of strength and confidence. Of course, your practitioner will be closely involved, but the greater your level of participation, the better off you will be.

The first step in finding a physician is to figure out what you're looking for. Do you want a medical doctor? Does your insurance cover alternative practitioners? Does it matter if you see a man or a woman? These are questions you can ask yourself before beginning your search.

On the issue of conventional versus alternative care, you may decide you want to have a medical doctor as well as an alternative practitioner who is knowledgeable about natural therapies. It's okay to seek the services of more than one health care professional, as long as each knows what the other is doing.

If you're concerned about how your doctor will react to your decision to pursue alternative remedies, keep in mind that attitudes about such approaches are changing rapidly within allopathic medicine. Medical schools and the American Medical Association are strongly encouraging medical doctors to ask patients if they are using natural remedies, and to be respectful if they are. In fact, the practice of complementary medicine—combining conventional and alternative treatments—has grown tremendously since the 1990s. Moreover, studies in medical journals have confirmed an increased willingness by medical doctors to make referrals to alternative practitioners.

Part of the reason for this shift is that doctors don't want to alienate their patients. But many medical doctors also realize that they have something to learn from other health fields and that this information can be used compatibly with conventional care. Of course, there are still those who dismiss alternative therapies. If your current doctor falls into this category, you may want to consider looking elsewhere. It's crucial to have a doctor you can be honest with and who respects your right to make decisions about your health care. Even if you have different views on certain things, the ideal situation is for both of you to accept these differences and work together as a team.

One obstacle you may face is insurance. While many health plans now pay for certain kinds of alternative care, the reimbursements are usually not comparable to those for conventional treatment. Health maintenance organizations (HMOs) and preferred provider organizations (PPOs) typically offer even less choice. If you are restricted by your coverage and find that you can't be in full partnership with your doctor, don't forget that you are still in charge. Demand as much information as possible, and request referrals or second opinions if you're not satisfied with your care.

Many alternative practitioners are aware that their services are largely limited to the affluent, and there's some effort to change that, both individually and collectively. Some naturopathic clinics, for example, offer a sliding billing scale based on ability to pay. One factor to consider is that, although out-of-pocket payments to alternative physicians may be an imposition, the long-term cost of natural medicine may ultimately be less than that of conventional care. That is, by taking more responsibility for their health, those who seek out alternative care tend to get sick less often and spend less money on expensive prescription drugs and high-tech surgical procedures.

In looking for an alternative practitioner, you will encounter a wide range of choices. Doctors of Oriental medicine, naturopaths, osteopaths, homeopaths, herbalists, Ayurvedic physicians who practice Indian medicine, acupuncturists, chiropractors—all of these and more can be found in most major cities, and in many smaller ones as well. There is also an increasing number of medical doctors who have some training in alternative therapies and incorporate them into their practice. You may decide that you want to consult with more than one alternative practitioner, although it's best not to go overboard. And while it's fine to combine some of the different therapies—for example, nutrition, yoga, acupuncture, and herbs—make sure that these approaches complement one another.

While critics of natural medicine use scare tactics about quacks and frauds, it does pay to do some checking. In contrast to medical doctors, who are regulated consistently, alternative practitioners are held to varying standards. Whether you're dealing with a conventional or alternative physician, it pays to ask lots of questions. Find out as much as you can about their training and experience. If you can't get a satisfactory answer, move on.

One of the best ways to find a practitioner is to ask your friends, family members, and colleagues for a recommendation. Keep in mind, however, that a lot depends on chemistry and personal taste. The person you choose should feel right to you, and you alone. Most importantly, remember that you are the employer, and that it's your body.

Questions to Ask When Looking for a Doctor

Health care practitioners, like others you hire for professional services, work for you. Therefore, you want to know what you're getting before you sign on the dotted line. The best way to make sure is to ask plenty of questions. Here are some of the basic issues to discuss:

- What are your views on fertility enhancement and infertility?
- Do you believe in preventive therapies?
- How important do you think diet is to conception, and are you able to work with me on improving my nutrition?
- What are your beliefs regarding natural medicines such as herbs, aromatherapy, flower medicines, acupuncture, and homeopathy?
- Do you support the use of mind/body techniques to reduce stress?
- Do you have any background or training in complementary medicine?
- Are you comfortable with patients who pursue these therapies?
- Can I reach you easily if I have questions?

Assuming that the answers are satisfactory, be very direct about your need to work together. If the practitioner seems to have any qualms about such an approach, you should probably look for someone else.

Introducing the Program

Clearing space in your life, making a commitment to yourself, and finding a good doctor are all essential to a natural fertility plan. Once you've done these things, you're ready to begin. Here are the elements of the Six-Step Natural Fertility Program.

Step 1: Track Your Ovulation

Chapter 5 features the first step in the program, and perhaps the most important information you will need to know. You will be instructed on how to take your basal body temperature (BBT) and examine your cervical mucus, and how to chart this information in order to recognize your ovulatory pattern. This step is crucial, since once the egg has left the ovary it generally has only 24 hours in which it can be fertilized.

You will develop and keep a fertility journal that will track not only ovulation but the treatments you and your practitioner choose. By using the journal, you and your partner will better understand how to undertake the program and increase your chances of successful conception.

Step 2: Follow the Dietary and Nutritional Supplementation Guidelines

What you put into your body really does count, especially if you want to get in shape for conception. For this reason, the diet and supplementation facet of our program is one of the most important. In order to enhance fertility, you have to cut out the worst elements and add the best. Most of us just don't eat as well as we should. Our crops are sprayed with pesticides, grown in depleted soil, and sprayed with polluted water; the beef and poultry we eat are full of growth hormones; the fish we consume is often loaded with mercury or other dangerous pollutants.

Unfortunately, many couples examine their diet only after unsuccessful attempts at conception. Yet there are many foods that can strengthen the body and prepare it for pregnancy. Chapter 6 will discuss the global issues surrounding diet, such as eating a whole-foods diet and avoiding foods (such as nonorganic dairy or meats) with artificial hormones. We'll look at how foods can boost health and vitality, and provide ideas for integrating them into your diet. Foods with specific benefits for fertility will be outlined, as well as foods to avoid.

Many women are either underweight or overweight. Chapter 6 will provide strategies for dealing with these issues, such as suggesting that you work with your practitioner to ensure that a proper diet is being followed.

New studies on supplementation show that they can drastically improve a couple's chance of conception. The B vitamins, vitamin C, vitamin E, and zinc, among other nutrients, are all critical for reproductive health. Chapter 6 will offer recommendations on how to boost your fertility through vitamin and mineral supplementation.

Step 3: Use Herbs, Aromatherapy, Flower Remedies, and Other Natural Therapies to Boost Fertility

Due to an increased awareness and acceptance of complementary therapies, natural healing approaches are increasingly being integrated into American health care. Among the most popular are herbal medicine and two closely related fields: aromatherapy and flower remedies. Homeopathy and acupuncture are also being embraced by many people.

Chapter 7 will look at how these therapies can enhance fertility. While aromatherapy and flower remedies can be safely used at home, you will be instructed to use herbs only with the assistance of a trained medical practitioner.

Step 4: Integrate Exercise, Movement Therapies, and Massage into Your Routine

When the endocrine system is working at its best, the endorphins it produces through exercise, movement, and massage foster a sense of well-being that can actually assist the body during the conception process. Not only do these natural opiates aid in balancing already delicate hormones, but endorphins encourage a sense of mental and emotional well-being that can help reduce stress.

Chapter 8 will discuss specific examples of movement therapies that have multiple benefits, such as yoga, chi gung, and tai chi, and how they can be used to strengthen the body and facilitate conception. We'll also examine how massage can help prepare your body for pregnancy, as well as foster intimacy between couples during the often stressful times when fertility issues arise.

Step 5: Use Mind/Body Techniques to Reduce Stress

An important study from Beth Israel Deaconess Medical Center in Boston showed that the stress of trying to have a baby can literally prevent couples from reaching their goal. In fact, we've all heard anecdotes about couples who finally give up trying to get pregnant—and then do. That's because the constant worrying and agonizing over fertility issues can actually produce increased amounts of stress hormones that suppress the immune system and block the circulation of blood flow and vital energy to the organs.

Chapter 9 will discuss various methods for reducing stress, including breathing exercises, visualization, meditation, and other self-relaxation techniques.

Step 6: Keep Your Sex Drive Active

Although this step may seem like the easiest component of the program, in reality it's not. Many couples find that the need to perform on demand takes the fun out of their lovemaking.

Chapter 10 will outline a variety of things that can be done to rev up your sex life, from weekend getaways to fantasies to different positions. We'll also list some natural therapies for stimulating intimacy, including foods and herbs that work as aphrodisiacs. In addition, we'll offer guidelines on what steps to take during and after sex to increase the chances of healthy conception.

Keeping a Fertility Journal

As you begin the process of enhancing your fertility, it will be helpful to start a journal. Keeping a diary not only will make it easier to follow the program but will provide an outlet for your thoughts and feelings as you adopt the changes outlined above.

If you've used journaling before, you probably know how beneficial it can be. Recording your daily experiences is one of the best ways to ground yourself, particularly during difficult or challenging times. After several weeks, you'll be able to read over your early entries and gain perspective on how the program is affecting your life.

Keeping a journal might sound like yet another commitment in an already hectic schedule. But all you need is 10 or 15 minutes in the evening. Chances are that within a short period you'll look forward to sitting down and reflecting on the day. Giving yourself enough time helps, as does finding a comfortable spot in your home to write.

Journaling is a forum for creativity, so feel free to come up with a format that works for you. Here are some basic guidelines that will help you get started.

Chart Your Symptoms

Depending on your particular situation, you may be experiencing physical or emotional symptoms related to your fertility. If so, keep a daily record of what they are and when they occur, noting any changes.

Chart Step 1: Keep Track of Your Ovulation

In Chapter 5, we'll explain how to tell when you're ovulating and provide a sample chart for recording key menstrual cycle markers. You can use your journal to elaborate on the physical aspect of this process, as well as to chronicle your feelings as you become more aware of your ovulation pattern.

Chart Step 2: Follow the Dietary and Nutritional Supplementation Guidelines

We are what we eat—but what is that? This is the place for you to keep tabs on your diet. Write down everything you eat and drink each day, answering each of these questions:

- What?
- When?
- How much?
- How did I feel while eating?
- How did I feel afterward?

Also write down what supplements you take, including the dose, and when.

Chart Step 3: Use Herbs, Aromatherapy, Flower Remedies, and Other Natural Therapies

Tracking your use of herbs and other natural therapies can help you discover how well they are working. Each day, write down the remedies you take or treatment you receive, along with symptoms you may have and whether they are improving.

Chart Step 4: Integrate Exercise, Movement Therapies, and Massage

You'll probably want to make an exercise schedule for yourself when you start the program. Here you can record your actual workouts and how they affect your physical and emotional health.

Chart Step 5: Use Mind/Body Medicine to Reduce Stress

As with exercise, stress-reduction techniques can have an immediate and noticeable impact on how you feel. Keep a log of the mind/body methods you use and the changes that follow.

Chart Step 6: Keep Your Sex Drive Active

Whether your lovemaking is great or needs improvement, it's important to stay in touch with what's working, or what's not. Write down the days you've made love, the details of what happened, and how you felt about it.

Again, a journal is very personal, so give yourself the freedom to experiment with style and content. Some women will only want to record the basic elements of the program, whereas others may be inspired to include lengthy descriptions of everything they are experiencing. Remember that there's no right or wrong way to keep a journal. Whatever form your journal takes, it will be a helpful part of a natural approach to fertility.

Getting Started

In the chapters that follow, each of the six steps already mentioned will be explained in detail. Of course, there's no guarantee that you will get pregnant by adhering to these guidelines. However, by using the program in partnership with your health care practitioner, you will improve your health and vitality and give yourself the best chance to conceive naturally.

CHAPTER FIVE

How to Tell When You're Ovulating

In the previous chapters, we've discussed what infertility actually means and why alternative approaches may be the best option to help you get pregnant. We've also looked at the various stages of the menstrual cycle, as well as conditions, both in women and men, that can affect fertility. Now you're ready for the first step in enhancing your fertility: learning how to tell when you're ovulating.

While it may sound relatively unsophisticated compared to high-tech fertility treatments, determining when you ovulate—and timing intercourse accordingly—can play a major part in helping you conceive. "Timing can make all the difference in the world in getting pregnant," says Suzann Gage, director of the West Hollywood, California–based Progressive Health Services, which specializes in women's health care. "Women are better able to identify the optimum time [to try and conceive] by learning through observation the specific changes that take place in their body and their cycle."

This chapter will show you how to detect ovulation and

your fertile days each month. You'll learn how to measure and interpret changes in both body temperature and cervical fluid, and how to keep track of these changes. You'll also learn how to time sexual activity according to fertility, how to detect possible ovulation problems, and how to make the process of monitoring your ovulation a positive part of your relationship and sexual life.

The Rebirth of Fertility Awareness

For thousands of years, women have used their knowledge of the fertility cycle either to avoid pregnancy or to conceive. Before the development of cheap, reliable contraceptives, fertility awareness was the primary means of birth control. Likewise, prior to the modern era of high-tech infertility treatments, women relied largely upon an understanding of their reproductive rhythms to get pregnant.

Over the past half-century, much of this knowledge has been lost with the professionalization of health care. As society has come to rely more and more on science and medical authorities, we have become increasingly out of touch with our bodies and how they work. For women, whose reproductive health has been left mostly to male doctors, this has created an aura of mystery around one of the most natural of human functions: conception.

Fortunately, the pendulum has now begun to swing back in the other direction. Women are once again learning to recognize their fertility signals and are putting this knowledge to use as they plan their families. At the same time, attitudes toward fertility awareness are changing in the medical profession as more practitioners realize its value. And scientific advances in reproductive medicine have added greatly to the understanding of fertility, leading to more accurate techniques for family planning.

Much of the credit for this shift goes to the women's movement, which understood that in order for women to become empowered, they had to gain greater control over their bodies. The feminist revolution that pushed for equality in the workplace and the home also led to major changes in women's health care. Beginning in the 1970s, women's health clinics started to become more widespread. These institutions have educated millions of women about their reproductive systems, helping them to plan or avoid pregnancy.

The explosive growth in alternative medicine has also contributed to the rebirth of fertility awareness and other natural ways of achieving conception. As we have sought to demystify our health care, we have rediscovered natural techniques such as ovulation detection. These methods are not only empowering but can be very effective.

Menstrual Chart Versus Fertility Chart

Before learning how to tell when you're ovulating, it's important to keep in mind the difference between a menstrual chart and an ovulation chart.

Many women keep a calendar of their menstrual cycle. It is useful in determining the average length between periods and can be helpful in anticipating symptoms associated with premenstrual syndrome (PMS). Charting ovulation, in contrast, can provide you with much more exact knowledge of your reproductive cycle. It takes a little more time than keeping a basic menstrual calendar, but the rewards can be great.

A menstrual calendar simply notes when bleeding begins and ends each month. An ovulation chart, by contrast, covers the changes that occur during your entire cycle—from menstruation to preovulation to release of the egg to the thickening of the uterine lining.

Following this process day by day will allow you to tell with much more precision when your egg will move from the ovaries to the uterus. This in turn will guide you in trying to fertilize the egg.

For some women, becoming aware of their ovulation cycle and putting that information to use is all that's necessary to overcome difficulties in getting pregnant. Even for those who require other measures, however, understanding fertility patterns can play an important role in achieving the goal of conception.

The Basic Signs: Cervical Mucus, Basal Body Temperature, and Luteinizing Hormone

There are several ways you can determine the approximate time of ovulation. All involve measuring the natural changes that take place as your menstrual cycle unfolds.

One key change is in the mucus produced by the cervix. Prior to ovulation, a woman starts to produce fertile mucus, which helps sperm to reach the unfertilized egg. After ovulation, a different kind of cervical mucus is present. The difference is apparent by changes in texture, appearance, and smell.

Another telltale sign is an increase in basal body temperature (BBT), or waking temperature. This rise is caused by heightening levels of progesterone. Shortly after a woman ovulates (or in some cases, just before), her temperature will go up anywhere from 0.6° to 0.8°. It will remain at an elevated level until her period arrives.

Ovulation can also be detected by changes in a substance called LH, or luteinizing hormone (see Chapter 2). Prior to ovulation, there's a dramatic increase in the level of LH. To monitor this rise, you can purchase a special home-test kit that measures the amount of LH in the urine.

Checking Your Cervical Mucus

Whereas a rise in BBT lets you know that ovulation has just occurred, changes in the mucus produced by your cervix tell you that ovulation is imminent. Learning how to recognize these changes can be an invaluable tool in achieving conception.

Just as women's menstrual cycles vary, the quantity, appearance, smell, and feel of cervical mucus is different from woman to woman. With this variation in mind, here is a general description of the various stages of the menstrual cycle and the corresponding changes in cervical mucus.

Postperiod For several days after you stop bleeding, the cervix does not produce any mucus. During this time, there usually will be no vaginal discharge.

Preovulation The cervix starts to produce a sticky mucus, some of which is discharged from the vagina. This mucus gradually becomes creamier and more slippery.

Around ovulation A few days before ovulation, the mucus becomes clearer, feels thinner, and may drip noticeably from your vagina. At this point it is similar in consistency to egg whites. In addition, it may have a sweet taste and odor. This is fertile mucus, in which sperm can survive for several days. Fertile mucus is structured so that sperm can move easily through it and advance toward the fallopian tubes. It may last until a day or two after ovulation.

Postovulation After several days of egg-white mucus, the cervix starts to produce a thicker, stickier, often salty-tasting variety, and continues to do so until your next period. This mucus is not conception-friendly, blocking the passage of sperm.

During the course of your cycle, you can keep track of the changes in your cervical mucus and record them on your BBT chart. This will help you recognize your ovulation pattern and identify your fertile days.

How to Identify Fertile Mucus

Knowing when you are producing fertile mucus is one of the keys to enhancing fertility through ovulation detection. Once you can tell fertile mucus from nonfertile mucus, you'll know when to time intercourse to increase the chances of conception.

There are various ways to check the progression of your cervical mucus during the ovulation cycle. While some women may be able to detect fertile mucus by inspecting the discharge on their underwear or a piece of toilet paper, the most reliable method is to place a finger inside your vagina and examine the mucus.

How can you tell for sure if it's fertile? Most women will find that their mucus becomes thinner, wetter, and more slippery. According to Gage, however, the stretch test is your best guide. "It can be really thick or really thin and watery. It can be crystal clear or slightly opaque or yellowish or even pink. The key difference is that when you pick fertile mucus up, you can get it to form a thread between your fingers, the same way you can get egg whites to stretch between your fingers."

Gage notes that the amount and duration of fertile secretions can vary considerably. Some women produce very little and stop after a day, whereas others produce much larger quantities for a week or more. She adds that many women produce secretions that contain both fertile and nonfertile mucus. "As long as fertile secretions are there, you're fertile."

One simple way to improve the sperm-carrying capacity of cervical mucus is to take a teaspoon or two of Robitussin cough medicine just prior to your fertile days. Robitussin not only thins mucus in the lungs, it also can thin cervical mucus, making the mucus more conducive to sperm.

Cervical mucus secretions can be affected by various factors including birth-control pills, vaginal infections, sexually transmitted diseases, and certain vaginal products. Swimming, showering, bathing, and unprotected intercourse can also alter cervical mucus for several hours. If you have an infection or a sexually transmitted disease (STD), have recently been on the pill, or are using a vaginal product, checking your cervical mucus is not an effective way to monitor ovulation.

Checking Your Basal Body Temperature

Charting your resting body temperature is another effective way to help you keep tabs on your ovulation pattern. The key here is accuracy and consistency.

Either a glass or a digital thermometer can be used to measure BBT. Some women prefer a digital instrument, as it's much quicker. A digital oral thermometer can be placed in the mouth, in the vagina, or under the armpit, although once you've chosen a location you should stay with it throughout your cycle. (To use the armpit technique, put the thermometer directly on the skin in the center of your armpit and fold your arm across it.) When you hear a beep, look at the reading and mark it down on your BBT chart (see page 89). It's okay if you forget to mark it right away, as the reading will be saved by a memory function.

Although the digital thermometer can be very convenient, some women find it easier to use a glass thermometer. "The trouble with the digital thermometer is that you have to insert it at exactly the same angle every time," says Gage. "You can be thrown off."

A standard glass thermometer will work, but it's best to get a special BBT thermometer because it has readings of 0.1°. The glass thermometer can also be placed in the mouth, in the vagina, or under the armpit. Insert the thermometer for 5 to 10 minutes, then read the temperature and record it on your BBT chart. The glass thermometer will also preserve the reading if you don't mark it down immediately.

Keep in mind that in order to get an accurate reading, you

have to take your temperature as soon as you wake up. If you get up and walk around for a few minutes, or even just lie in bed, a BBT chart will not work. "Your temperature starts to rise as soon as you're awake," says Gage. "This is where difficulties come in for some women. They get too high a reading."

If you follow this routine for several months, a pattern should appear. Once you know approximately when you ovulate each month based on a rise in BBT, you can time intercourse to maximize the likelihood of pregnancy.

It's very important to remember that the BBT method should be used to plan the following month's attempts at conception rather than the current month's, since the rise in temperature comes near the end of a woman's window of fertility. Timing intercourse to the day when your temperature increases may not substantially improve your chances of getting pregnant.

Another thing to consider is that a slight *decrease* in temperature prior to the sustained increase might be the ovulatory sign you're looking for. "For some women it's the bottom-most point that's most closely associated with release of the egg," says Gage. "We have known women who were using BBT and were trying to get pregnant after their temperature went up and weren't getting pregnant. Then they started charting their cervical mucus and noticed that first their os [cervical opening] closed, then their temperature went up a day or so after that, meaning that the temperature was low when the egg popped out. We urge women to compare their basal body temperature chart to their cervical mucus chart, because that has proven to be a much more accurate indicator."

As with cervical mucus, certain factors can prevent accurate BBT readings. First, as mentioned above, you must measure your temperature at the same time each day. Also keep in mind that infections, colds, and even stress can result in elevated body temperature, thereby giving a distorted picture of your overall cycle.

Using the Luteinizing Hormone Kit

A third option for determining ovulation is the LH kit. You can purchase the kit at a pharmacy and test your urine for the presence of LH.

Each kit contains either sticks or a pad that reacts to your urine, along with a chart to keep track of each day's measurement. The presence of any LH in the urine is indicated by blue. When levels increase, a darker shade of blue will appear, which means that ovulation will follow in 12 to 36 hours.

The LH kit can be somewhat time-consuming as well as costly. And, according to Gage, it doesn't always give an accurate picture of when a woman is ovulating.

"We've had a number of women tell us they tried the LH kits and weren't getting pregnant, then they started looking at their cervix and saw that the kit wasn't lining up with what their body was telling them. Some women find they line up well; others don't." She adds that sometimes they turn color a little early or late. "We urge women to compare [the LH readings] to what their cervical secretions are telling them."

Other Ways to Detect Ovulation

Changes in basal body temperature, cervical mucus, and LH are the three primary indicators of ovulation. But there are other symptoms that may be helpful in recognizing your unique ovulation pattern.

One of these is the consistency of the cervix. You can learn to feel the difference in cervical texture by squatting and then inserting a finger into your vagina as far as possible. After your period, your cervix will feel tight and hard. As ovulation approaches, it will become soft and wet, and the opening, or os, will widen to allow sperm to travel through. You'll also notice that the cervix is higher in the vagina and harder to reach at this time. After ovulation, the cervix returns to its prior consistency and position. (With women who have already had a vaginal birth, the cervix always remains somewhat open.)

Another sign of ovulation is changes in the texture of saliva, which mimics the cervical mucus. These changes can be detected with a special home-testing kit that includes slides and a microscopic lens with which to view the saliva or cervical mucus samples. A pattern of straight lines on the slide indicates that the fertile phase of the cycle is underway.

Several other symptoms are sometimes associated with ovulation, including breast tenderness, light bleeding, increased sexual desire, rashes, and pelvic pain (often called *mittelschmerz*). These are less reliable markers, however, and should not be used as the primary method of determining ovulation.

Using a Speculum to Check Your Mucus and Cervix

One way to more closely follow the changes that take place during your ovulatory cycle is to watch those changes with your own eyes. This can be done easily with a speculum, a device that allows women to see inside their vagina and observe the cervix. Your physician will instruct you on how best to use it.

As ovulation approaches, the opening to the cervix, known as the os, widens. At the same time, glands in the cervical canal produce fertile mucus in response to stimulation from maturing ovarian follicles.

With a speculum, you can observe your cervix and see how it changes. You can also see where cervical mucus comes from and monitor the transition from the nonfertile to the fertile variety.

Here's how to use a speculum to watch the changes in your cervix and mucus:

1. Put a clean towel on the bed.
2. Recline on the bed with your legs spread wide.
3. Insert the speculum like a tampon and open the handle.
4. Using a hand mirror, shine a light inside your vagina.
5. Look for your cervix at the bottom of your vagina.

Gage has shown thousands of women how to do self-observation and says it's easy with a little practice. "Most women find it doesn't take very long. They often become very familiar with what their cervix looks like and can spot changes in an instant," says Gage.

Gage encourages women who are trying to conceive to become familiar with their cervix. "We have found that observing changes in the cervix seems to be more precise in timing for most women, even compared to BBT, and definitely the LH kit."

Which Method Is Most Accurate?

Every woman must decide for herself which method she prefers to monitor ovulation. Time, convenience, and comfort are all issues to be considered. For many women, though, the highest priority is accuracy.

If done carefully, tracking cervical mucus provides a very precise picture of the ovulation process. Most importantly, it lets you know when you are fertile. According to one study that looked at numerous ways of determining ovulation, this method was the most accurate for pinpointing women's fertile days each month.

Checking basal body temperature is also a very reliable way to calculate ovulation. It is somewhat less useful, however, as the sole means of trying to get pregnant through ovulation detection. This is because the increase in temperature comes only *after* ovulation, when the monthly window of fertility is almost closed. However, for women with a very regular cycle, a BBT chart can serve as an effective way to plan sexual intercourse each month to coincide with their fertile days.

The LH kit offers another option for monitoring ovulation, and in many cases it works well. However, because of the time and expense involved, some women will not find it as practical. Others may learn that tracking their LH surge, while helpful, does not by itself allow them to identify their fertile days as accurately as other methods.

Women who are willing and able to commit significant time and effort to fertility awareness may want to monitor BBT, cervical mucus, and other symptoms. This is known as the symptothermal approach. By combining these methods, you can both establish your general ovulatory pattern (BBT) and gauge when you are fertile during any given month (cervical mucus).

The least accurate means of establishing the time of ovulation is the calendar method—commonly known as the rhythm method. This approach is based on the average length of a woman's cycle. Since the second phase of the cycle is generally fixed at 14 days, ovulation is calculated by subtracting 14 from the total number of days between periods. Sexual intercourse is then timed to coincide with the week or so prior to the presumed day of ovulation.

The problem with this approach is that many women's menstrual cycles vary in length from month to month. Using the calendar method thus leaves too much to chance. Though it's better than nothing, it is not recommended for women who want to get the most out of fertility awareness.

When to Have Sexual Intercourse

Now you know how to monitor your unique ovulation pattern according to changes in your body. The next step is to coordinate sexual intercourse (or insemination) with your window of fertility.

Pregnancy depends on the presence of live sperm and a viable egg. Sperm can survive for up to 5 days in the vagina, although the average life span is 3 days. An egg can generally be fertilized for about 24 hours after ovulation. Thus, most women are fertile for a week or less during each menstrual cycle.

Some women have more fertile days per cycle than others. This is mostly tied to how many days a woman produces fertile mucus. It's also possible for an egg to survive for as long as 3 days, which can extend the number of fertile days in a cycle.

To maximize the possibility of conception, you and your partner should have regular intercourse beginning a week or so before ovulation and continuing until 1 or 2 days afterward. Since it takes 24 to 48 hours to replenish the sperm supply after ejaculation, having sexual intercourse every other day during this period is just as effective as daily intercourse.

What to Expect from Fertility Awareness

Knowing how to determine ovulation and timing sexual intercourse accordingly does not, of course, guarantee that you will become pregnant. But it can be an important part of a natural approach to fertility, and in some cases it can significantly shorten the time spent trying to conceive.

Medical research has demonstrated the benefits of fertility awareness. One study of women using fertility awareness techniques showed that among those who had never conceived, 80.9% became pregnant in the first cycle, compared to 22% to

30% of women in the general population. (For women who had been pregnant before, the figure was 71.4%.) By the end of the fourth cycle, 100% had become pregnant.

This study included women with normal fertility, meaning the ability to get pregnant within 6 months. But the ovulation method has also proven effective among women having trouble getting pregnant. Joseph Stanford, M.D., who specializes in natural family planning, reports that 20% to 40% of patients referred to the Natural Family Planning Center in Omaha, Nebraska, are able to conceive within 6 months by using the ovulation method.

Other Benefits of Fertility Awareness

Monitoring basal body temperature and cervical mucus can help increase your chances of getting pregnant. But it can also help you recognize ovulatory problems and seek out appropriate treatment.

As noted previously, you will typically experience an increase in BBT at ovulation. If this does not occur, it may be an indication that you are not ovulating. If the temperature rise is not sustained throughout the rest of your cycle, a hormonal imbalance may be present that could affect your ability to conceive.

Likewise, cervical mucus production should follow the progression already described. If you are not producing the stretchy, egg-white-like mucus, this may also be a signal that you are not ovulating.

One symptom associated with ovulatory problems is an irregular period. Although the length of your menstrual cycle may change as you get older, significant fluctuations within a short span are often correlated with irregular ovulation. Also be aware that even if you're bleeding, you may not be ovulating.

Beyond helping you recognize ovulatory problems, fertility awareness offers another potential benefit: increased sexual intimacy. Monitoring the ovulatory cycle and timing sexual intercourse to it requires discipline and commitment. Couples willing to make this commitment often find themselves talking in ways they never have before about sex. This can be a valuable tool in heightening sexual intimacy, particularly for those already experiencing difficulty in getting pregnant. The communication and teamwork that go along with fertility awareness can help couples cope with the emotional strains of trying to conceive.

"Couples who use fertility awareness effectively throughout their reproductive lives experience no side effects and often find an increased intimacy in their relationships, which includes a shared responsibility for their combined fertility," observes Christiane Northrup, M.D., author of the acclaimed book *Women's Bodies, Women's Wisdom.*

Feeling Comfortable with Ovulation Detection

Monitoring BBT and cervical mucus might seem cumbersome at first, but most women are able to master these techniques. A bigger obstacle may be overcoming inhibitions.

In a society where health care has been so professionalized, few women are accustomed to taking an active role in monitoring their reproductive functions. Thus, checking basal body temperature or examining cervical mucus may initially be off-putting for some women. The same is true of talking about ovulatory cycles and windows of fertility with your partner.

Such inhibitions are natural and should not discourage you. Remember that fertility awareness requires a strong commitment to self-care and a high level of communication between partners. And give yourself some time to become comfortable with the process.

Getting Help in Getting Started

Seeking professional advice can be extremely helpful for couples who choose to use natural family planning techniques. The same is true for those who decide to use fertility awareness to facilitate pregnancy.

Introducing fertility consciousness into the whole area of sexuality and working with it daily is a pretty new concept for many," writes Dr. Northrup. Noting that personalized instruction can address various issues encountered by those new to fertility awareness, she adds, "The quality of a woman's (or couple's) experience . . . often depends upon the quality of instruction given and follow-up care received."

Trained health care workers can offer several kinds of assistance. First, they can explain in clear, simple language how to use various fertility awareness techniques. Second, they can provide reassurance to couples who are skeptical or wary of the process. They can also refer couples to other medical resources if necessary. Family planning clinics can be found in most cities (see Resources) and usually offer sliding-scale fee arrangements.

1. Write the date of your first period and circle it.
2. Cross off every day your period continues.
3. Do the same for the next month(s).
4. *Don't worry* if your period doesn't run like clockwork. Every woman has her own menstrual clock.

Sunday	Monday	Tuesday	Wednesday	Thursday	Friday	Saturday

Sunday	Monday	Tuesday	Wednesday	Thursday	Friday	Saturday

Sunday	Monday	Tuesday	Wednesday	Thursday	Friday	Saturday

Sunday	Monday	Tuesday	Wednesday	Thursday	Friday	Saturday

Sunday	Monday	Tuesday	Wednesday	Thursday	Friday	Saturday

Sunday	Monday	Tuesday	Wednesday	Thursday	Friday	Saturday

GUIDELINES FOR AN ACCURATE BASAL BODY TEMPERATURE (BBT) CHART

1. The first day of your menstrual flow is day 1 of your BBT chart. Do *not* include spotting prior to your period as day 1. Your temperature should drop when your menstrual flow starts. Record your temperature every day, both when you are menstruating and when you are not. This information is important.

2. Make sure you note the actual day of the month in the space provided on your chart.

3. Use an oral, digital, basal body thermometer only. A regular thermometer won't do!

4. Take your temperature each morning before you get out of bed. Place the thermometer under your tongue, in your vagina, or under your armpit for at least 2 to 3 minutes.

5. Don't eat, drink, or smoke before you take your temperature.

6. Record your temperature by using a dot, not an X or a checkmark.

7. Use a down-pointing arrow to indicate the days you had intercourse.

8. Record any premenstrual symptoms if there is space on the chart. Otherwise, use your symptom chart to help link a certain temperature to a symptom.

9. Note special considerations such as illness or fever.

10. Change charts when you get your period again.

Finally, on one of your charts, record what you're eating, how much you're exercising, and whether you're under any unusual stress. Coffee, alcohol, dieting and exercise, and emotional stress all affect your menstrual cycle. By cutting out certain foods or vices, you can see if your menstrual cycle changes.

Sunday	Monday	Tuesday	Wednesday	Thursday	Friday	Saturday

Sunday	Monday	Tuesday	Wednesday	Thursday	Friday	Saturday

Sunday	Monday	Tuesday	Wednesday	Thursday	Friday	Saturday

Sunday	Monday	Tuesday	Wednesday	Thursday	Friday	Saturday

Sunday	Monday	Tuesday	Wednesday	Thursday	Friday	Saturday

Sunday	Monday	Tuesday	Wednesday	Thursday	Friday	Saturday

CHAPTER SIX

Eating and Supplementation for Natural Conception

Since the 1970s, the connection between what we eat and how healthy we are has become apparent to both the medical community and the public. As attitudes have shifted about the importance of diet to all aspects of our physical and psychological well-being, health care practitioners have increasingly stressed the role of nutrition in contributing to a healthy pregnancy. Prenatal nutrition has become a standard part of medical practice, and dozens of books and countless articles have been written on what women should eat to ensure a healthy baby.

Less emphasis, however, has been placed on how eating impacts conception itself. While this is starting to change, the fact remains that diet and supplementation are often ignored by those in the fertility field. Thousands of couples struggling to have a child thus pursue expensive, invasive, and time-consuming methods without ever taking stock of how poor eating habits, along with the use of such substances as caffeine, alcohol, and tobacco, may be compromising their ability to have a child.

In this chapter, we will show how diet can be a major factor in enhancing your fertility. We'll discuss the benefits of a whole-foods diet and offer advice about what foods to eat and which ones to avoid. We'll also look at how weight can affect your efforts to get pregnant and help you determine the best way to achieve a weight that's conception-friendly. Finally, we'll provide guidelines for a supplementation plan that will ensure you receive the nutrition you need for optimum fertility.

The Whole-Foods Diet

Despite increased awareness of how improper eating affects health, the typical diet for many people is filled with highly processed foods weak in nutritional value. "The American or Western diet today is replete with inadequacies of micronutrients and major imbalances," says Steven Bailey, N.D., of Portland, Oregon.

Poor eating habits translate into poor health. Diets high in fats, simple sugars, highly processed food, pesticides, chemicals, and preservatives lead to a range of illnesses and diseases. It stands to reason that people who consume fewer of these substances while emphasizing whole foods rich in nutrients enjoy better health. A whole-foods diet features a broad spectrum of foods, including grains, legumes, fruits, vegetables, raw seeds and nuts, and lean or low-fat animal products.

Why is a whole-foods diet so important for promoting pregnancy? One reason, says Dr. Bailey, is that the four primary female hormones involved in reproduction—follicular hormone, luteinizing hormone, estrogen, and progesterone—are produced by the body from products we get in the diet. More generally, organ health depends on the body's ability to repair damaged tissue, which it does through nutrients found in food. "If there is an inadequacy or imbalance in the diet, these systems are not going to work as effectively," explains Dr. Bailey. He adds that a whole-foods diet will also improve digestion and liver function, both important components of reproductive health (see "Digestion and Elimination," later in this chapter).

By giving us more nutritional value, whole foods can improve health and even reverse symptoms of illness. For women who have followed various diets and eaten erratically over the years, switching to a whole-foods diet may seem like a huge challenge. But making the transition is very manageable if you take it slowly. Eventually, you'll find that whole foods taste better, fill you up more completely, increase your energy, and provide a greater sense of well-being.

Any dietary change requires patience as well as a sense of balance. Don't try to eliminate every "bad" food; focus instead on making good choices most of the time. As you start to enjoy the health benefits of a whole-foods diet, you'll probably find that a periodic high-fat splurge is all you will desire.

While a whole-foods diet will emphasize certain foods and minimize others, there is no one plan that's right for everybody. In his practice, Dr. Bailey has found that few patients will stick to a rigidly planned diet. Instead, he outlines the basic principles of a whole-foods regimen, then gives them a blank food diary and later evaluates it for general balance.

Here are some guidelines, outlined in *Alternative Medicine: The Definitive Guide*, that will help you achieve nutritional balance through diet:

● *Eat more fiber.* Fiber is essential to a well-functioning digestive system, which plays a critical role in reproductive health (see "Digestion and Elimination," later in this chapter).

"I've seen a lot of my patients with slow bowel transit times, where it takes many days for food to be eliminated from the body. When this happens, many breakdown products are absorbed into the system, impairing optimal health of the uterus and liver," says Dr. Bailey.

Good sources of fiber include fruits, vegetables, and whole grains. You can measure the amount of fiber you are eating by looking at your stools, which should be soft, well formed, and easily passed. If your diet doesn't provide enough fiber, helpful additives include wheat bran flakes or psyllium seed husks (a heaping teaspoonful before or with meals). Fiber works best taken with lots of water and supplemented by gentle exercise, such as walking, which encourages intestinal motility.

• *Consume less fat.* Adequate body fat is essential for conception. Most people, however, get far more fat than they need, and will improve both their overall health and their fertility by reducing fat intake.

Following a whole-foods diet will achieve this goal, since the percentage of total calories from fat in most vegetables is less than 10%, and is 16% to 20% in most grains. These numbers are dwarfed by the fat levels found in animal products: whole milk and cheese, for example, derive 74% of their calories from fat, while a rib roast's percentage of calories from fat is 75%.

Fat should account for 25 to 30% of your total daily calories. If you consume an average of 2100 calories a day, that would mean 630 fat calories (or 70 grams).

Reducing fat can be beneficial for women who may need to lose weight in order to enhance their fertility. Women who are already underweight or have low body fat may need to increase their consumption of fat, but they should strive to get it from the healthiest sources (see "Good Fat, Bad Fat," later in this chapter).

• *Decrease sugar consumption.* Those sugar products may taste good, but you probably already know that they represent empty, nutritionally bankrupt calories. More than that, high sugar intake can lead to hypoglycemia, which may affect reproductive hormonal balance.

The first things to limit are foods made with such sweeteners as white sugar, brown sugar, and high-fructose corn syrup. This includes most candy, cakes, pastries, soft drinks, ice cream, and yogurt. Also be aware of the sugar content in cereals, crackers, jams and jellies, salad dressings, condiments, juices, and other nondessert items. When possible, opt for foods sweetened with maple syrup, molasses, rice syrup, barley malt, or fruit juice—all of which are higher in nutrient value than simple sugars and are metabolized more slowly by the body.

● *Increase variety.* Many of us are creatures of habit when it comes to diet, yet there are good reasons to diversify. Different nutrients are found in different foods, and a well-balanced diet will contain a wide variety of vegetables, grains, cereals, and nuts. Dr. Bailey notes that the typical diet today contains far fewer food species than in the past. When choosing fruits and vegetables, think like a painter preparing a palette and select a multicolored array of produce. This will optimize your nutrient intake.

● *Eat lower on the food chain.* Humans may have a strong carnivorous streak, but curbing your consumption of animal products is a good way to enhance your health. Part of the reason is that most beef, poultry, fish, and dairy products are filled with pesticides, hormones, and chemicals. Animal foods also tend to be high in fat. These drawbacks can be substantially reduced if you make a habit of eating lean, organic meats and low-fat dairy products.

Even the most conscientious animal-food lover should strive to consume more plant-based foods. Grains, nuts, seeds, legumes, fruits, and vegetables offer an abundance of nutrients that enhance fertility as well as overall health.

Adequate protein is essential, of course. You should consume about 70 grams a day. But there are numerous nonanimal foods rich in protein. These include soy products, legumes, nuts, and seeds. Keep in mind that some women process nonanimal proteins better than others, and that your diet should reflect your body's own specific needs (see "Vegetarians and Fertility," later in this chapter).

• *Go organic.* Organic foods are not just a fad. Produce grown without chemical fertilizers, pesticides, and herbicides have much higher nutrient value. Similarly, animals that are raised on organic feed and not given antibiotics and hormones make for healthier meats.

As often as possible, buy foods that have been produced free of chemicals. It is easy to begin by purchasing organically grown whole grains and beans available in most natural food stores. Some organic vegetables are commonly found in many grocery stores as well.

Switching to primarily organic produce is more costly, but it offers real benefits. Buying organic meat products is also important. "The highest intake of pesticide comes from feedlot red meat and dairy," notes Dr. Bailey. He adds that studies have shown that pesticides mimic estrogen and occupy estrogen receptor sites in the body.

Be wary of foods bearing the label "natural," which can be very misleading. Many foods produced with chemicals, antibiotics, and hormones are dubbed "natural" by manufacturers. With animal foods, a "natural" label only guarantees that the animals weren't given any antibiotics or hormones in the 2 weeks prior to slaughter. If you have to choose between naturally and commercially raised animal foods, natural is better, but your best choice is organic.

● *Drink plenty of fluids.* Liquids are an important component of good health. And water is the best. "Most liquids—sodas, coffee, milk—are not providing significant hydration," notes Dr. Bailey. Along with purified water, diluted juices and herbal tea can also be added to your fluid repertoire.

A Guide to Fertility Foods

Following a whole-foods diet will ensure that you are getting good nutrition for both overall health and fertility. Here are some of the foods that can maintain and strengthen the reproductive system (see "Nutrients and Fertility," later in this chapter, for more details).

Grains

Benefit   Good sources of vitamin E, B vitamins, and trace minerals, which are all vital to reproductive health.

Source   Wheat germ, whole wheat, rye, buckwheat, brown rice, millet, cornmeal, oatmeal, whole-grain pastas.

Beans

Benefit   Soy beans are known to help with hormonal balance. Other beans provide a good stable sugar source both before and during pregnancy.

Source   Soy, navy, black, adzuki, chickpea, lentil, pinto, kidney.

Vegetables

Benefit   High in carotenes, which are important for cell division. Good sources of folic acid, essential fats, and antioxidants, all of which play key roles in fertility. Vegetable enzymes are vital to removing toxins from the body and also facilitate healthy circulation.

Source   Fresh vegetables, especially yams, winter squash, sweet potatoes, carrots, bok choy, asparagus, Chinese napa cabbage, mushrooms, dark leafy greens (kale, collards, and turnip greens), green peppers, burdock, beets and beet greens, tomatoes, black-eyed peas, romaine lettuce, broccoli, cabbage, parsley, black radishes, fennel.

Sea Vegetables

Benefit   Excellent source of trace minerals essential for reproduction, especially iodine, which is needed for healthy thyroid function. Thyroid irregularities are associated with hormonal and ovulatory problems.

Source   Kelp, seaweed, blue-green algae.

Fruits

Benefit   High in antioxidants, which reduce toxins in the body and thus help prepare the body for healthy pregnancy. Also a key source of fiber, which aids in digestion and elimination and thus enhances fertility (see "Digestion and Elimination," later in this chapter).

Source   Fresh and dried fruits, including citrus fruits, black currants, bananas, figs, avocados, apples, plantains, cherries, apricots, cantaloupe, berries, pomegranates, white part of fruit rinds.

Raw Seeds and Nuts

Benefit   Seeds are one of the richest dietary sources of essential fats, which are critical to hormonal balance as well as cell membrane and neurological development. Nuts are high in fertility-friendly vitamin E.

Source   Almonds, walnuts, chestnuts, hazelnuts, cashews, pecans, Brazil nuts, sunflower seeds, sesame seeds, pumpkin seeds.

Fish

Benefit   Excellent source of protein, which is crucial to reproductive function, and essential fatty acids.

Source Salmon, sardines, mackerel, herring, tuna, trout, oysters, shrimp, clam, roe, lobster, halibut.

Poultry and Meats

Benefit Strong source of protein.
   Source Free-range organic beef, chicken, lamb, pork.

Dairy Products

Benefit High in protein and calcium.
   Source Low-fat milk and yogurt, cheese, eggs.

Fats and Oils

Benefit Certain oils are high in essential fatty acids.
   Source Cold-pressed virgin olive oil and sunflower oil, flaxseed oil, cod liver oil, unrefined sesame oil, unsalted butter.

Beverages

Benefit Liquids act to remove toxins from the bloodstream, thus helping to avoid digestion and elimination problems that can compromise fertility.
   Source Filtered water; fresh, diluted juice; herbal tea; grain coffee substitute.

GOOD FAT, BAD FAT

Fats come in three varieties: monounsaturated, polyunsaturated, and saturated. While the body requires some of each, the healthiest kind is monounsaturated, followed by polyunsaturated, and then saturated. Here's a simple guide that will help you make good choices when it comes to fat consumption.

Monounsaturated Fats Found in olive oil and canola oil, these fats increase low-density lipoproteins (LDL), or good cholesterol, while lowering high-density lipoproteins (HDL), or bad cholesterol.

Polyunsaturated Fats   Safflower, sunflower, and corn oils are good sources of polyunsaturated fats, which contain fertility-friendly essential fatty acids.

Saturated Fats   Animal foods and tropical oils such as coconut and palm oil are the main sources of saturated fats, which at high levels have been linked to heart disease. Some saturated fat is necessary, however, for cholesterol production.

Nutrients and Fertility

Adopting a whole-foods diet will put you on the right track toward getting the nutrition you need for conception. Here is a basic guide to how vitamins and minerals contribute to a woman's fertility, and the best food sources for each of them.

Vitamin A

Function   All DNA (deoxyribonucleic acid) replication is vitamin A dependent. Vitamin A is important for hormone production, as well as for digestion and elimination, which can both affect fertility. *Caution:* Excessive amounts while pregnant can lead to birth defects.

Source   Fish; milk; egg yolks; green, red, and yellow vegetables and fruits.

Vitamin B$_1$ (Thiamin)

Function   Vital for proper metabolism, thus helping to ensure adequate nutrition for the reproductive system.

Source   Whole grains, nuts, seeds, dried beans, lean pork.

Vitamin B$_2$ (Riboflavin)

Function   Critical to thyroid function, which is necessary for menstrual and ovulatory health.

Source   Milk, yogurt, cheese, fish, beef, eggs, avocados, mushrooms, fortified breads and cereals.

Vitamin B_3 (Niacin)

Function   Crucial for hormonal function, circulation, the nervous system, digestion, and conversion of fats and proteins into energy, all of which are needed for reproduction.

Source   Whole grains, legumes, soy beans, nuts, green vegetables, eggs, milk, fish, chicken, beef.

Vitamin B_6

Function   Essential for proper hormonal balance. A deficiency leads to an increase in estrogen and a decrease in progesterone, and can cause miscarriage. "We know that the activity of hormone replacement and estrogen activity is associated with B_6 and vitamin C functions," says Dr. Bailey. "They are generally recommended supplementally to women who are looking to improve fertility." B_6 can relieve premenstrual syndrome (PMS), and increased B_6 intake is necessary for women using oral contraceptives. *Caution:* Excessive amounts may cause nerve damage.

Source   Fish, chicken, beef, whole grains, legumes, carrots, potatoes, eggs, bananas.

Vitamin B_{12}

Function   Critical to red blood cell production and nervous system function. Insufficient B_{12} can result in anemia, which may prevent ovulation. Deficiency may be caused by malabsorption, inflammatory bowel disease, hydrogen chloride deficiency, a vegan diet, excessive antibiotics or anticonvulsives, or megadoses of vitamin C or copper. Must balance B_{12} with folic acid.

Source   Clams, salmon, lamb, lobster, tuna, cheese, milk, halibut, brewer's yeast, microalgaes (spirulina, blue-green algae).

Vitamin C

Function Plays a role in hormone production, is needed to assimilate iron, and helps maintain the integrity of the blood supply in the uterus and placenta to keep the egg implanted. *Caution:* Excessive amounts can interfere with ovulation.

Source Citrus, cruciferous vegetables, tomatoes, strawberries, blackberries, blueberries, cherries, green peppers.

Folic Acid

Function Deficiency may affect hormonal function. Insufficient folic acid can lead to a variety of birth defects, including neural tube defects and spina bifida. Cervical dysplasia is also associated with deficiency. Also be aware that use of oral contraceptives can result in depleted folic acid. Extra B_{12} should be taken with folic acid.

Source Dark green vegetables, legumes, nuts, chicken liver, brewer's yeast, orange juice, beef liver, black-eyed peas, romaine lettuce, cantaloupe, egg yolks.

Bioflavonoids

Function Increase blood flow and may help strengthen uterine lining, thereby decreasing chance of miscarriage.

Source Grapeseed extract, green tea, broccoli, cabbage, parsley, white part of fruit rinds.

Vitamin D

Function Deficiency may be linked to reproductive disorders. Vitamin D also regulates metabolism of calcium and phosphorus, which are both required for healthy hormonal function. Extended use of cortisone drugs and phenytoin (Dilantin) can cause deficiency. *Caution:* Excessive amounts can lead to birth defects.

Source Egg yolks, fortified milk, fortified cereals, salmon, tuna.

Vitamin E

Function A potent antioxidant important to oxygenation and balanced hormone production, vitamin E is generally associated with fertility. May help prevent miscarriage and ensure regular ovulation.

Source Wheat germ, sunflower seeds, almonds, pecans, hazelnuts, vegetable oils, leafy green vegetables.

Vitamin K

Function Needed for blood clotting, which is essential to both general and reproductive health.

Source Kale, Swiss chard, turnip greens, broccoli, alfalfa, brussels sprouts, cauliflower, cabbage, green tea.

Calcium

Function Deficiency can cause estrogen deficiency, resulting in ovulation problems. Also important for proper digestion and metabolism, which help maintain fertility.

Source Milk, cheese, yogurt, broccoli, collard greens, almonds.

Chromium

Function Needed for proper metabolism, which ensures adequate nutrition to the reproductive system.

Source Whole grains, brewer's yeast, potatoes, nuts, fish.

Copper

Function Aids body's use of iron, thereby preventing anemia, which can disrupt ovulation.

Source Shellfish, organ meats, nuts, legumes, whole grains, soy, peas, avocados, garlic, potatoes, tomatoes, bananas.

Iodine

Function   Crucial to thyroid function, which is necessary for menstrual and ovulatory health.

Source   Table salt, kelp, saltwater fish.

Iron

Function   Deficiency can cause anemia, thereby interfering with menstrual function and ovulation. Vitamin C helps the body absorb iron.

Source   Leafy green vegetables, liver, beef, shellfish, legumes, whole grains, potatoes, egg yolks, dried fruits, brewer's yeast, kelp, seeds, wheat bran.

Magnesium

Function   Important for estrogen production; helps correct unexplained infertility and prevent miscarriage.

Source   Nuts, legumes, whole grains, leafy dark green vegetables, milk, shellfish.

Manganese

Function   Aids in glucose utilization, enzyme activation, and cholesterol synthesis—all important to hormone production.

Source   Whole grains, nuts, leafy green vegetables, pineapple.

Phosphorus

Function   Important to the secretion of hormones, which is vital to ovulatory function.

Source   Milk, cheese, nuts, legumes, cereals, fish, chicken, beef.

Potassium

Function   Essential to healthy kidney and nerve function, both of which are needed for reproduction.

Source   Bananas, oranges, potatoes, beef, chicken, milk, yogurt.

Selenium

Function   Essential for thyroid function, which is necessary for menstrual and ovulatory health. Also lessens dietary and heavy metal toxicity, which can compromise fertility.

Source   Brazil nuts, fish, chicken, beef, oats, brown rice.

Zinc

Function   Needed for processing of genetic materials. A deficiency can impair the synthesis of follicle-stimulating hormone (FSH) and luteinizing hormone (LH) and interfere with thyroid function, disrupting the menstrual cycle and causing infertility as well as delivery problems and low-birth-weight babies. Inflammatory bowel disease, celiac disease, and alcoholism may result in deficiency, along with diuretics. "Zinc is very important," says Janet Zand, O.M.D., L.Ac., of Austin, Texas. "We always hear about zinc for the immune system. If a woman is not menstruating, she may be zinc deficient." *Caution:* Excessive amounts may lead to mineral imbalances that can compromise fertility.

Source   Fish, chicken, cheese, eggs, cereals, nuts, beans, wheat germ.

Essential Fatty Acids (EFAs)

Function   Critical for healthy hormone function and fertile mucus secretions, as well as immune function and tissue health. Omega-3 and omega-6 EFAs should be balanced, but most people get far more omega-6.

Source   Fish, soy beans, navy beans, kidney beans, pumpkin seeds; also flaxseed oil, evening primrose oil, borage seed oil, walnut oil, black currant oil (all high in omega-3 EFAs).

Lecithin and Choline

Function   Essential to cell wall integrity, both in the ovum and sperms and the ovaries and uterus in general. Also important for proper liver function, which aids in conception.

Source   Beans, egg yolks, peanuts, wheat germ, liver.

Foods to Avoid

Generally speaking, a well-balanced whole-foods diet will help you avoid "bad" foods that can delay or prevent conception. As you plan your diet, the following items should be avoided or consumed conservatively:

- White rice and refined flour (found in white bread, bagels, crackers, cookies)
- Canned baked beans
- Frozen and canned vegetables
- Canned fruits
- Commercially roasted nuts and seeds
- Fried chicken, luncheon meats, nonorganic liver
- Deep-fried fish and shellfish
- Refined sugars
- Refined and processed oils, margarine, hydrogenated oils
- Coffee (with and without caffeine), caffeinated teas, alcohol, sodas with phosphates (sugared and diet), sugared drinks

Other Substances to Avoid

Even the health-conscious person will have an occasional appetite for certain indulgences. For women trying to conceive, however, it's vital to understand the risks associated with various stimulants.

Caffeine   There's nothing like a cup of coffee or a piece of chocolate to pick you up. But if you're trying to get pregnant, these well-loved crutches and other caffeinated products can be a major letdown.

For women trying to get pregnant, the primary concern with caffeine is its effect on adrenaline, says Dr. Bailey. "Caffeine is known to prolong the life of adrenaline." This triggers the fight-or-flight syndrome, which can interfere with fertility. Dr. Bailey also notes that adrenaline diverts blood away from the digestive and reproductive systems, directing it instead to the muscles and brain. As caffeine consumption increases, proper functioning of the uterus and ovaries can be impaired and may even lead to miscarriage.

Research has found that caffeine is associated with significant delays in conception. One study showed that women who consumed more than 300 milligrams of caffeine daily were almost three times as likely not to get pregnant over the course of a year than women who had no caffeine. In another study, women who had more than 500 milligrams of caffeine a day— five cups of coffee—took 11% longer to get pregnant than those who had no caffeine in their diet.

Remember that significant amounts of caffeine are present not only in coffee but also in tea, cola, chocolate, and many nonprescription medications including some pain relievers. Here's a guide to common sources of caffeine:

Brewed Coffee (5-ounce cup): 60–180 milligrams

Instant Coffee (5-ounce cup): 30–120 milligrams

Black Tea (5-ounce cup, steeped): 25–77 milligrams

Iced Tea (12-ounce glass): 67–76 milligrams

Baker's Chocolate (1 ounce): 25 milligrams

Soft Drinks (12-ounce serving): 36–59 milligrams

Nonprescription Drugs: 30–200 milligrams

Prescription Drugs: 30–100 millligrams

Alcohol   It's almost universally known that drinking during certain stages of pregnancy is a definite no. Over the last several years, research has also shown that alcohol can decrease fertility.

One study involving a group of 430 Danish couples found that women who consumed 1 to 5 drinks a week had a harder time getting pregnant than those who abstained. Women who had 10 or more drinks a week were one third as likely to conceive as those who didn't drink at all. Another study at the Johns Hopkins School of Medicine in Baltimore found that even one glass of wine a month can have a dramatic effect on fertility.

There is some debate over whether an occasional drink poses a significant risk to conception. In *Getting Pregnant: What Couples Need to Know Right Now*, Niels H. Lauersen, M.D., suggests limiting alcohol intake for at least 1 month before attempting pregnancy. For those who are having problems conceiving or have a history of miscarriage, he recommends avoiding all alcohol for at least 48 hours prior to intercourse. Researchers think that alcohol may lower progesterone levels, making it difficult for an egg to successfully be implanted in the uterus.

Tobacco   Tobacco has destructive effects on numerous aspects of human health, and fertility is no exception. Hundreds of studies have been conducted on the effects of tobacco on conception, pregnancy, and childbirth. The results offer a grim picture.

Not only does smoking make it harder to conceive, it also greatly increases the chances of miscarriage. For women smokers who do give birth, their babies stand a greater chance of having low birth weight and experiencing various health problems. Dr. Bailey notes that smoking increases calcification of the placenta, impairing oxygen delivery.

Marijuana   Another substance to avoid before and during pregnancy is marijuana, which has been linked to both miscarriage and fetal growth problems.

Other Recreational Drugs   Not surprisingly, drugs such as cocaine, LSD, PCP, and heroin can cause a host of serious problems, from miscarriage to premature birth to birth defects. The rule of thumb is to stay away from all street drugs before and during pregnancy.

Vegetarians and Fertility

A well-balanced vegetarian diet, either with or without dairy products, can provide a good nutritional foundation for pregnancy. Women who eat milk and eggs but do not consume beef, chicken, pork, and fish generally do not have a problem with adequate protein intake. Those who avoid all animal foods can get sufficient protein from soy products, legumes, nuts, and seeds, but they must be sure to be disciplined in their eating habits.

Not all women are ideal candidates for a diet without animal protein. "You need to get enough protein to support a pregnancy," says Katherine Zieman, N.D., L.M., of Portland, Oregon, who says 60 to 90 grams a day is required. "With women who don't eat animal protein, it's a matter of if they can metabolize enough plant protein. If not, they get thin, and without enough body fat, you won't conceive."

A vegetarian diet high in carbohydrates can be an obstacle to conception. Women who do not eat any form of animal protein should consume large quantities of soy products and legumes, along with a wide range of vegetables and fresh fruits. Vegetarians (particularly nondairy vegetarians) may be deficient in zinc, iron, vitamin B_{12}, and folic acid, all of which can be increased through supplements.

If you're a vegetarian, the best approach is to consult with your practitioner and discuss your diet in detail to determine whether it's giving you the nutrition you need to get pregnant.

Digestion and Elimination

In preparing their patients for pregnancy, many alternative practitioners focus on an area often ignored by their counterparts in conventional medicine: digestion. This approach is based on a very sound premise: the body must be able to digest food properly in order to supply adequate nutrition to the reproductive organs. "Digestive integrity is a very important concern, and absorption and delivery function are very important to having a healthy reproductive system," states Dr. Bailey. Close attention is also paid to elimination, which plays an important role in reproductive health.

Susan Lange, O.M.D., L.Ac., co-director of the Meridian Center in Santa Monica, California, uses a cleansing program for women who want to conceive as part of a comprehensive prepregnancy program. "I want people to clear up some of their issues before they get pregnant," says Dr. Lange.

Healthy functioning of the liver and kidney, along with the spleen and pancreas, is essential to optimize fertility. "To have healthy egg and sperm, the kidney energy, the liver energy, and the spleen/pancreas energy have to be strong," explains Dr. Lange. "They are responsible for fertility—for healthy hormones and conception. That is why I focus on digestion. My goal is to get those organs healthy, and the rest of the body will start to follow suit."

Elimination is equally important, she says. "If elimination isn't good, you get a backlog from the large intestine into the small intestine, and through the walls of the bowels back into the bloodstream." When this happens, the blood returns to the liver, which then has to process the same level of toxins repeatedly. As a result, the liver and kidneys get overburdened.

Compromised liver and kidney function can affect such crucial elements of reproduction as hormonal balance and nutrient supply to the uterus. Symptoms of an overburdened liver include PMS, large menstrual clots, headaches, very irritable constipation, or diarrhea around menstruation, says Dr. Lange. Kidney deficiency may manifest itself in very light periods and fatigue during menstruation.

Often, the culprit in poor digestion and elimination is gut damage, which can have a variety of causes, such as the overuse of antibiotics and stress. The stomach, explains Dr. Lange, becomes like a murky swamp of various toxins. "When that happens, the body becomes unable to digest properly, it can't break down the food, and the woman doesn't get nourished."

Toxins in the gut can leak into the uterus, says Dr. Lange, sometimes resulting in low-grade infections that can impair fertility. "If the good bacteria are being killed off and the bad ones are proliferating, there can be low-grade infection going on in the pelvis."

Since environmental and dietary toxins are virtually impossible to avoid, it's important to maintain healthy digestion and elimination so that the body can handle the load. "If the gut is healthy, those toxins get flushed out, they don't leak so much into the liver and kidneys," says Dr. Lange. "If the toxins do leak, the liver and kidneys can handle it." As an example, she cites how people react differently to mercury, which can cause liver damage and thereby lead to infertility. "Those who are affected by this are the ones whose elimination organs are overwhelmed."

Dr. Lange recommends a 90-day cleansing program before trying to conceive. She puts her patients on a prepregnancy herbal cleanse designed to assist the elimination organs in clearing out pesticides, stimulate the intestines, build muscle tone, help rid the body of chronic infection, and balance the hormones. Foods such as meat and dairy are to be eaten in smaller amounts, while vegetables, fruits, and grains are increased. She emphasizes that such a program is not to be undertaken during pregnancy.

Supplementation

Ideally, we would get all of the nutrients we need from the foods we eat. For one, vitamins and minerals are most easily absorbed by the body in their natural form. Equally important is the fact that striving for maximum nutrition through a well-balanced diet is the best way to ensure overall health.

For most of us, though, some help from nutritional supplements is a sensible idea. As a result of the depletion of our soil, even the most health-conscious people have difficulty getting adequate nutrition solely through food.

Multivitamins and other supplements should never be used as a substitute for a healthy diet, but they can fill in the gaps that inevitably occur. "The more highly processed foods are in the diet, the more absolutely important it is to get good supplementation to offset empty calories," says Dr. Bailey.

There are many good multivitamins on the market today. One important rule to bear in mind is that one-a-day multivitamins, while convenient, don't provide as much nutrient value as those that must be taken several times daily. It's impossible to pack enough usable nutrition into one tablet, explains Dr. Zieman.

Elizabeth Burch, N.D., recommends the following supplement dosages for women before they try to conceive:

Vitamin A: 5000 international units

Vitamin B$_1$: 1.5 milligrams

Vitamin B$_2$: 1.6 milligrams

Vitamin B_3: 17 milligrams

Vitamin B_6: 2.2 milligrams

Vitamin B_{12}: 2.2 micrograms

Folic Acid: 800 micrograms

Vitamin C: 500–1000 milligrams

Vitamin D: 400 international units

Vitamin E: 400 international units

Vitamin K: 65 micrograms

Calcium: 1200 micrograms

Magnesium: 500 milligrams

Iron: 30 milligrams

Phosphorus: 1200 milligrams

Iodine: 175 micrograms

Selenium: 65 micrograms

Adequate levels of zinc are also important to conception. Dr. Burch suggests 12 milligrams a day, along with 2 milligrams of copper and 100 micrograms of chromium. Dr. Burch notes that women should not take more than 5000 units of vitamin A once they're pregnant.

For women coming off birth-control pills, special supplementation is suggested. Dr. Stephen Davies and Dr. Alan Stewart recommend the following dosages:

Vitamins B_1, B_2, B_3: 10–50 milligrams each

Vitamins B_5, B_6: 50–100 milligrams each

Vitamin B_{12}: 200–400 micrograms

Vitamin C: 250–2000 milligrams (or more)

Folic Acid: 400 micrograms to 2 milligrams

Vitamin E: 50–200 international units

Magnesium: 100–200 milligrams (or more)

Zinc: 5–15 milligrams (or more)

Manganese: 3–5 milligrams

Iron: depends on whether a deficiency is present

Inositol: 50–75 milligrams

Choline: 50–75 milligrams

Weight and Fertility

For many women, weight is a complex, often emotional issue. From an early age, girls are bombarded with messages and images telling them what they should look like. In response, too many form unhealthy eating habits that can have serious physical and psychological repercussions.

A woman's fertility can be greatly affected by body weight. Underweight women, particularly those with insufficient body fat, are prone to menstrual irregularities that can interfere with ovulation, thus preventing conception. Women who are excessively overweight also have a harder time getting pregnant, as obesity can disrupt menstruation as well as impair normal hormonal function.

A study conducted at the University of Washington found a dramatic correlation between weight and infertility. Women who were 20% or more above their ideal weight were almost five times more likely to have trouble conceiving. Women who were 15% or more below their ideal weight ran a similar risk.

In another study done by German researchers, a group of 35 obese women who had been unable to conceive were put on a weight-loss program. After decreasing their weight by an average of almost 20 pounds, 10 of the women became pregnant, and 8 delivered healthy babies. Weight loss among obese women also decreases the chance of miscarriage.

Eating disorders can increase the chances of infertility. Conditions such as anorexia and bulimia deprive the body of essential nutrition, often disrupting a woman's menstrual cycle. One study found that nearly 17% of the subjects experiencing infertility also had eating disorders.

You don't have to conform to popular norms of beauty and fitness to get pregnant. But it's important to understand that there is a weight range for optimizing the chances of conception. Dr. Lauersen offers the following weight guidelines for women trying to conceive:

Height	Weight (pounds)
4'10"	109–121
4'11"	111–123
5'0"	113–126
5'1"	115–129
5'2"	118–132
5'3"	121–135
5'4"	124–138
5'5"	127–141
5'6"	130–144
5'7"	133–147
5'8"	136–150
5'9"	139–153
5'10"	142–156
5'11"	145–159
6'0"	148–162

Dr. Lauersen notes that women with small bones—that is, a wrist measurement of 5½ inches or less or an ankle measurement of 8 inches or less—should use the lower end of the weight range. Those with a wrist measurement greater than 6 inches or an ankle measurement greater than 9 inches should use the higher end of the scale.

Dr. Lauersen emphasizes that while staying within these guidelines is important, levels of body fat must also be taken into account. Body fat can be determined through testing or can be calculated by using a body mass index (BMI), which you can find out how to do in many nutrition books.

Although exercise is an important part of a healthy lifestyle, excessive levels can be detrimental for women trying to get pregnant (see Chapter 8). When body fat drops below a certain level, menstruation and cervical mucus production are often adversely affected, making conception more difficult.

For women who need to lose weight, the first thing to check is the thyroid, says Dr. Zieman, noting that hypothyroidism often causes ovulation problems and miscarriage. The next step is to fill out a diet diary and start making changes. The best approach takes into account various factors and tries to minimize the need for unhealthy food choices. "If you need candy, why? Were you depressed, tired? How can you alter your lifestyle so you don't have that problem? What kind of herbs can we use as a pick-me-up?"

In addition to modifying diet, Dr. Zieman encourages women to make exercise a part of their daily routine by doing such things as parking a bit farther from the office and walking to and from work. "I start to work with people on walking. I never make them start an exercise program—it's too hard. I try to find out what in their life they can change and incorporate exercise into everyday life." Dr. Janet Zand notes that a number of supplements can be helpful in losing weight, including evening primrose oil and flaxseed oil, the amino acid l-carnitine, and chromium picolinate.

SUCCESS STORIES

Dr. Bailey has used dietary changes, along with other treatments, to help many women who were having difficulty getting pregnant. Here he recounts the story of one patient:

She and her husband had been going to fertility clinics for probably 5 years. They had insurance that covered 80%, and they had still spent $30,000 and had not been successful. I gave them a diet diary and suggested some fairly major changes, from highly processed, low-fiber foods to more crunchy vegetables, essential fat supplements, and a high-quality vitamin/mineral. I also used a homeopathic remedy called *Causticum* and did some counseling. . . . And I did some spinal manipulation to increase circulation to the lower back.

About a month into the case, the woman became pregnant. She continued supplements and dietary changes and gave birth to a healthy child and now has had two children. The total cost was $500.

Should You Consult a Practitioner?

Healthy eating may seem simple, but getting adequate nutrition can be a real challenge. While it's important to educate yourself and take control of your diet, consulting with a trained professional can be extremely helpful in making the changes you need to optimize your fertility. A practitioner can evaluate your eating habits in the broader context of your reproductive and overall health and make practical suggestions for a fertility-friendly diet. Together, you can create a positive approach to eating that meets your nutritional needs.

CHAPTER SEVEN

Herbal Therapy, Aromatherapy, Flower Remedies, and Other Natural Healing Systems

Chapter 6 established how a healthy diet and nutritional supplementation can serve as a strong foundation for enhancing fertility. These steps often work best in combination with one or more holistic therapies.

Herbal medicine, an ancient system of health maintenance with a long history in the treatment of infertility, is frequently used to complement changes in eating habits. Acupuncture is another venerable healing method and is commonly applied to fertility problems in conjunction with both nutritional and herbal therapy, particularly by practitioners of traditional Chinese medicine.

Two other approaches closely related to herbal medicine—aromatherapy and Bach flower remedies—have proven effective in strengthening female reproductive health. A third, the natural medicine known as homeopathy, can also help prepare a woman for successful conception.

This chapter will look at all of these increasingly popular

therapies. It will provide you with a basic understanding of how they work, discuss how each can contribute to optimal fertility, and highlight examples of women who have used them to become pregnant naturally.

A Note about Self-Care Versus Professional Care

One of the advantages of many natural fertility therapies is that they can empower you with the knowledge to take an active part in getting pregnant. In some cases, this means using self-care remedies, whereas in others it involves working closely with a practitioner.

Several of the therapies described below can be administered at home. Aromatherapy and flower remedies, in particular, lend themselves to self-care. In most cases, homeopathic remedies can also be safely taken without the supervision of a practitioner, although professional guidance is often useful.

Herbal medicine requires more caution. Although some herbal remedies are perfectly safe, others have mild to serious side effects. Many herbs are contraindicated for certain conditions, including pregnancy. Another factor is the proliferation of brands with their varying forms and dosages, which can make it difficult to know what to buy. For these reasons, we advise that you consult with a practitioner before taking herbal remedies.

Herbal Medicine

Although only recently starting to find mainstream acceptance in North America, herbal medicine is one of the oldest systems of healing known to humankind. Used for thousands of years by Asian civilizations, it remains the most widespread form of medical treatment on the planet. Herbs also serve as one of the foundations for Western health care, providing the source material for many prescription drugs.

Herbal remedies are derived from various plant parts, such as the flower, leaf, root, or stem. They can be used to treat a broad spectrum of health conditions and fall into nearly 20 categories, such as anti-inflammatories, astringents, stimulants, and tonics.

While herbs contain potent medicinal qualities, they tend to work more slowly and gently than their pharmaceutical counterparts. They can be taken in a variety of forms: capsules, tablets, extracts, tinctures, infusions, decoctions, oils, ointments, and so on. One of the most common preparations is herbal teas, which are consumed for enjoyment but also have multiple healing properties.

A trained herbalist can be an invaluable ally in guiding you through the world of herbal medicine. Herbalists are trained to select from among hundreds of possible remedies and often combine several herbs into a single formula.

Diagnosis

When treating a new patient, an herbalist will first diagnose the problem using techniques similar to those employed by conventional doctors, including a history, physical exam, and blood work, if necessary. For women who are having difficulty conceiving, Jill Stansbury, N.D., of Battle Ground, Washington, will first determine if the patient is ovulating and check the sperm count of her partner. She might also test hormonal levels and rule out inflammatory diseases, such as ovarian cysts and uterine fibroids, that can prevent implantation of the egg.

In addition, Dr. Stansbury, who chairs the Botanical Medicine Department at the National College of Naturopathic Medicine in Portland, Oregon, will also look for clues in the woman's general health. "Is there poor immune function and lots of infections, is there fatigue, is there hormonal insufficiency in the thyroid and adrenal glands, is there poor nutritional status or heavy metal toxicity, are there menstrual irregularities? Each one would be treated individually."

Janet Zand, O.M.D., LAc., of Austin, Texas, notes that herbal medicine is more effective for certain conditions than others, and stresses the importance of an accurate diagnosis. "I think that herbal medicine works best for a woman who has been to a doctor who says there's nothing wrong with you, go home and relax, or a woman who has tried a lot of medications and they haven't worked and doctors feel there's a hormonal problem, but the woman is not responding to conventional hormonal therapy. If a woman has a blocked fallopian tube, herbal medicine is not where to start. Much of my success through the years has come from knowing which patients to treat and which to send to a surgeon."

Strengthening the Reproductive System

Herbal medicine has long been used to enhance fertility. Like many natural therapies, it is usually most effective when combined with other remedies. "There are herbs that are really strong, but others are a tonic or foundational remedy that will cross over with nutritional or supplemental therapy," says Steven Bailey, N.D., of Portland, Oregon.

Herbal remedies can contribute to overall reproductive health as well as treat specific fertility-related ailments. Dr. Bailey has used herbal medicine for a range of conditions, including heavy menstrual bleeding and various premenstrual syndrome (PMS) symptoms. Although such problems do not always affect fertility, restoring a normal menstrual cycle can often be a critical step in preparing for healthy conception.

Dr. Bailey has found that some of the gentler herbs are highly effective in treating common menstrual complaints that may be related to fertility problems. For cramping, he recommends raspberry leaf tea. Pennyroyal and mint teas improve blood flow to the uterus and may be helpful in increasing the odds of conception, though these remedies should not be used during pregnancy as they can actually lead to miscarriage (raspberry leaf tea can be safely consumed before and after conception).

For severe cramps, Dr. Stansbury prescribes antispasmodic herbs such as cramp bark or wild yams. Although serious menstrual cramping is not unusual, she points out that in some cases it may indicate that conception is occurring but that the woman is spontaneously aborting because of uterine irritability.

Another menstrual disorder is periods that come every 2 or 3 weeks. This can make ovulation hard to detect or can indicate a hormonal abnormality, says Dr. Stansbury. She has found that chastetree berry may help restore a normal cycle.

Menorrhagia, or long-term bleeding, can be relieved with two common herbs: cinnamon and ginger. Both work exceptionally well, says Dr. Bailey, noting that cinnamon is best used in a tincture form and that ginger powder and apple juice can relieve heavy postpartum bleeding. Another remedy for menorrhagia is cayenne, which should be taken in capsule form.

For hormonal balance, Dr. Bailey suggests several herbal preparations, including dong quai, black cohosh, and partridge berry leaf. All three are good tonics for normalizing and improving the reproductive system, and should be used together with vitamins E and B$_6$. Two other herbs that help regulate the hormones are damiana (avoid during pregnancy) and wild yams.

To balance a woman's hormones, Dr. Zand often uses a dong quai formula during the first part of a patient's cycle, then changes to a wild yam preparation. "On the last day of her period, say from the 5th day to the 14th day of her cycle, I have a woman use some kind of dong quai combination," she explains. "From the 14th day until the beginning of her period,

I have her use some kind of wild yam preparation. So you're getting the estrogenic phase and then the progesterone phase. That will most always regulate the hormonal cycle."

Dr. Stansbury finds that hormonal imbalances often manifest themselves in symptoms such as breast tenderness, fybercystic breast disease, severe mood swings, and irritability. In order to normalize hormones, she emphasizes the importance of supporting the liver. "It's the liver that metabolizes and excretes hormones and gives feedback to the brain on what hormones are present," says Dr. Stansbury. "If we use herbs that regulate the liver, it tends to provide hormonal balance and give the brain the correct feedback." She recommends milk thistle along with many of the classic bitter roots such as burdock, dandelion, and yellow dock.

Herbal Remedies for Infertility

Herbs have wide-ranging applications in the treatment of infertility. According to Y. C. Chiang, O.M.D., Ph.D., of El Cerrito, California, herbal remedies can:

- Regulate imbalances between the liver and kidney functions, which can cause irregular menstruation, ovulation
- Increase circulation of chi, or energy, to treat irregular menstruation
- Expel accumulation of wetness and get rid of phlegm that may cause irregular ovulation
- Eliminate uterine infections that affect fertility
- Eliminate vaginitis, which "exhausts the fluid of the reproductive system" and slows down the mobility of sperm
- Dissolve small cysts and fibroids in the reproductive system that may cause infertility

There are dozens of herbal remedies that can help optimize your reproductive health and set the stage for healthy pregnancy. Below are many of the conditions associated with infertility and the herbs that are used to treat them.

Ovulatory Problems

Dr. Zand says the first step is to make sure the ovaries are in good shape by ruling out ovarian cysts and other serious conditions. She will then often prescribe evening primrose oil and a Chinese formula called hsiaoyaowan. She also uses various dong quai combinations.

Dr. Stansbury has found chastetree berry to be helpful in treating women who are not ovulating or who are ovulating irregularly.

Amenorrhea

Dr. Zand recommends a dong quai combination, and also uses royal jelly. She stresses that zinc deficiency is often responsible for amenorrhea, and that liquid B vitamin and vitamin E are also beneficial. According to Dr. Stansbury, chastetree berry can also be effective in restoring menstruation.

Cervical Mucus Disorder

Dr. Zand suggests a dong quai formula, along with vitamin E, zinc, and general good nutrition.

The Pill

For women coming off the pill, Dr. Zand recommends a dong quai formula, along with vitamin E and essential fatty acids.

Endometriosis

This disease, a common cause of infertility, can be difficult to treat. Dr. Stansbury recommends trying to reduce estrogen levels. This can be done by improving liver function as well as avoiding such sources of estrogen as nonorganic meat, dairy, and wheat products. "It's a small amount, but it may be cumulative for some people," says Dr. Stansbury. "Many pesticides actually bind to estrogen receptors in the body and have effects like estrogen, leading to excessive estrogen stimulation in the tissues, cysts, fibroids, endometriosis, and prostate disease and lowered sperm counts in men."

She also suggests eating soy products, which contain isoflavones, and taking the herb dong quai, which has coumestans. Both isoflavones and coumestans, explains Dr. Stansbury, have estrogenic effects and can bind to estrogen receptors. But since they're much less potent than either innate estrogen or chemically ingested estrogen, they can actually lower estrogen levels by crowding out these other hormonal agents.

According to Dr. Zand, the Chinese herb carthamus persica helps relieve inflammation in the lower abdomen associated with endometriosis. She adds that butiao can ease abdominal cramping and menstrual pain brought on by the disease. Dr. Zand also suggests vitamin E, while emphasizing the importance of seeing a practitioner.

POLYCYSTIC OVARY SYNDROME

Liver support is important in treating this condition, says Dr. Stansbury. The ailment is often associated with anovulatory cycles, amenorrhea, and elevated testosterone. She often uses saw palmetto, which helps regulate testosterone levels in the body and acts as a tonic for the whole reproductive system.

Dr. Stansbury recalls the case of a woman with total amenorrhea resulting from polycystic ovaries. "First we got her menstruating again with chastetree berry, angelica, and saw palmetto. We also put her on a good diet. Once she began menstruating, she was able to conceive and hold a pregnancy."

PELVIC INFLAMMATORY DISEASE

To treat this condition, the underlying infection must be identified, says Dr. Zand. She has found carthamus persica to be helpful for patients with PID, and sometimes butiao.

FIBROIDS

These growths, when large enough, can interfere with fertility, says Dr. Stansbury. "I've seen a few people's fibroids reduced greatly so they could carry their pregnancy." She advises women to use liver-support herbs (milk thistle, burdock, dandelion) and to consume a diet high in fiber to improve the metabolism of estrogen.

MISCARRIAGE

Mother's cordiale is a remedy that's been used for hundreds of years to prevent miscarriage. Dr. Stansbury reports that it can be quite successful in helping women carry a fetus to term.

Dr. Zand says that miscarriage often responds to progesterone-type treatment. "In Chinese medicine we say it has to do with deficiency," explains Dr. Zand. "We try to build the woman up by using progesterone creams and a dong quai formula, along with essential fatty acids and vitamin E."

THYROID DISORDERS

Thyroid problems can interfere with conception. The level of thyroid hormone can be determined with a laboratory test, but Dr. Stansbury also looks for physical symptoms, noting that some people have borderline irregularities not always detected by this test. Symptoms include a chronic feeling of coldness, low body temperature, digestive problems (specifically constipation), dry skin, slow growth of hair and fingernails, and some difficulty in losing weight. Although taking the thyroid hormone is advisable in some cases, Dr. Stansbury believes that it's preferable to stimulate the body to make its own hormone. She often prescribes fucus, which is high in iodine (a substance found in the thyroid) as well as copper and zinc. She also uses thyroid gland, derived from organic bovine thyroid tissue, along with iodine.

For hypothyroid problems, Dr. Zand will rotate a dong quai combination with the Chinese formula hsiaoyaowan, using the dong quai during the first half of the cycle and the hsiaoyaowan during the second. She also has found kelp and other seaweeds, along with the amino acid tyrosine and the B vitamins, to be helpful.

ADRENAL DYSFUNCTION

Another contributing factor to fertility problems is adrenal problems. Symptoms include fatigue, poor stress tolerance, anxiety, low immune function, and poor memory and concentration. To regulate adrenal activity, Dr. Stansbury suggests ginseng and licorice.

TOXINS

Detoxifying the body of heavy-metal contaminants can enhance fertility. Frequent bouts of vaginitis, cervical infections, or yeast infections may indicate that these toxins are present in significant amounts. Dr. Stansbury first advises that patients follow a diet high in fruits, vegetables, and fiber and low in sugar or refined flour products that break down easily into sugar, which feeds yeast. She also uses caprylic acid, an essential fatty acid that stops the reproductive process of yeast, as well as culinary herbs such as oregano, rosemary, and thyme, all of which are antifungal agents. Acidophilus is another well-known remedy for yeast infections. Other treatments, notes Dr. Stansbury, include preparations applied vaginally, such as boric acid, vinegar diluted with water, calengela, sage, and tea tree.

EMOTIONAL INSTABILITY

Depression, stress, and anxiety can be major factors in both general health deficiencies and fertility problems. Herbal medicine offers a number of remedies that can help alleviate these conditions. St.-John's-wort and SAMe have recently become popular as mood enhancers. Other common remedies include skullcap, kava kava, valerian, and vervain.

Herbs and Infertility—A Quick Reference

Here is a list of some of the most common herbal remedies used for infertility and their applications.

Chasteberry   Dr. Stansbury states that chasteberry can facilitate ovulation by triggering the production of luteinizing hormone and has been known to normalize menstruation in some women with amenorrhea.

Dong Quai   A popular herb for menstrual symptoms, dong quai is also beneficial in balancing reproductive hormones and strengthening the uterus, according to Dr. Stansbury.

Red Clover Blossoms   This herb is recommended by Dr. Stansbury for women who are low in estrogen, as it contains elements that act similarly to this vital reproductive hormone.

Licorice   Women with irregular periods and hormonal imbalance involving excess testosterone and insufficient estrogen may benefit from licorice, according to Dr. Stansbury.

Motherwort   This calming agent has been used for centuries to enhance fertility. It's particularly effective for women who are tired or worn out, and can help relieve menstrual problems.

True Unicorn Root   This herb stimulates the uterus and can be useful for women who experience miscarriage as a result of uterine weakness.

Ginseng   There are various kinds of this popular herb, including Siberian, American, and Korean (or Panax). Dr. Stansbury suggests ginseng both as a general tonic and as an aid in the regulation of reproductive hormones. "In Chinese medicine it's a chi tonic. To make a baby, you must have vital force. Ginseng helps improve vitality and immune function, and has steroidally active compounds for hormonal balancing. It's especially good if people seem to be deficient in some way—exhausted, getting lots of infections, having difficulty sleeping."

Red Raspberry   A classic uterine tonic, this herb has historically been used by women prone to miscarriage. Dr. Zand adds that red raspberry can be very effective in easing delivery, particularly if used regularly during the last trimester.

Stinging Nettle   Dr. Zand says that nettle is a great blood builder and makes a woman less susceptible to anemia. However, it should not be used by women who are pregnant, as it can lead to uterine contractions.

Burdock   This herb boosts estrogen production.

Black Cohosh   It stimulates the pituitary to improve ovarian function, according to Dr. Stansbury.

Alfalfa   Alfalfa has an estrogenic effect and thus can be helpful as a hormonal balancer.

Kelp   According to Dr. Zand, kelp can be useful in cases of infertility linked to low–normal thyroid function if the condition is responsive to iodine.

Ho Shou Wu   This herb can regulate ovulation and corpus luteum formation. It can also boost sperm count in men, says Dr. Zand.

Damiana   Both women and men with low sexual desire may benefit from damiana.

Blessed Thistle   This herb is used for hormone balancing and menstrual problems.

Liquid Chlorophyll   This supplement improves the quality of blood, says Dr. Zand. It can help purify the liver and regulate menstruation.

Gotu Kola   This herb is a good hormone balancer.

Sarsaparilla   This herb can function as a hormonal tonic. According to Dr. Zand, it has a mild testosterone effect and may be effective for women with low sexual desire.

Wild Yam   One of the most useful herbs for infertility, wild yam has a progesteronic impact, helping a woman to hold a pregnancy.

Herbs for Stress   St.-John's-wort, kava kava, valerian, vervain, skullcap.

SUCCESS STORIES

A woman in her mid-20s came to see Dr. Zand for infertility. She had been a competitive gymnast and had a history of anorexia. The woman was menstruating only two or three times a year. "Her doctor tried many different hormonal therapies, and her menstruation did not regulate itself," says Dr. Zand. "I treated her with a dong quai formula and acupuncture for 3 or 4 months. By the fifth month, she was pregnant." The treatment also included B vitamins, zinc, essential fatty acids, and a digestive enzyme.

A couple sought out Dr. Bailey after trying a wide array of techniques ranging from fertility drugs to frozen eggs that were fertilized and reimplanted. The woman had become pregnant several times but in each instance had suffered a miscarriage. Dr. Bailey put her on a regimen that included herbal yam products, glandular therapy, dietary changes, and nutritional supplementation. Within 3 or 4 months she got pregnant naturally and had a healthy natural birth.

Should You See a Professional?

Herbal medicine can be practiced safely without direct medical supervision, but only up to a point. Mild menstrual problems such as minor bleeding and cramping, for example, often can be relieved with over-the-counter herbal formulas.

It's important, however, not to underestimate the potency of herbal remedies. "Just because it's an herb doesn't mean it can't be toxic," cautions Dr. Bailey. He cites ephedra, which has been banned in competitive sports due to its heart-rate-elevating properties.

As noted previously, certain herbs pose a danger during pregnancy. Another concern with self-care is that you may misdiagnose a problem, leaving a potentially harmful ailment untreated. "Self-care may be appropriate, but only after enough work to make sure there isn't a serious underlying condition," advises Dr. Bailey. He adds that while it may be difficult to find a qualified herbalist or naturopath in many geographical areas, it's still best to consult a doctor to rule out major illness before embarking on a course of self-care.

Aromatherapy

While the name of this healing method may conjure images of New Age retreats, in truth it is a powerful branch of herbal medicine with wide applications. Used as far back as ancient Egypt, aromatherapy utilizes plant oils in various forms to treat everything from infections to arthritis to herpes. In addition, this holistic modality is known for its pleasurable, stress-relieving properties.

Aromatherapy remedies derive their therapeutic strength from naturally occurring chemicals that work on both the physiological and the emotional levels. When the aroma from an essential oil reaches the brain's limbic system, it can trigger changes in heart rate, blood pressure, stress levels, and hormonal activity. Essential oils are usually applied topically, although they can also be inhaled with the aid of a diffusor or added to bath water.

Diagnosis

Each of the essential oils in the aromatherapy pharmacy can be used for a range of conditions. Although remedies are often self-prescribed by matching them to a particular health problem, practitioners who use aromatherapy will conduct a thorough interview with a patient, noting all relevant physical and emotional symptoms.

Aromatherapy Remedies for Infertility

While aromatherapy is generally not used as a primary treatment for infertility, many of the essential oils have qualities that can enhance a natural approach to conception. They include the following:

Clary Sage   This oil helps balance hormones and improve circulation.

Sage   Like a number of oils, sage can raise estrogen levels.

Calendula   A cleansing oil, calendula supports the immune system.

Chamomile   This oil supports digestive function, which is important for conception, and also has a calming effect.

Geranium   Another hormone balancer, geranium calms the nerves.

Rose   This oil can boost fertility by regulating the blood and acting as a liver tonic. Rose should not be used during pregnancy, as it can bring on menstruation.

Ylang-ylang   This Chinese oil balances the nerves and can reduce sexual dysfunction.

Fennel, cypress, melliluca, and quinquinervia are also commonly used for low estrogen levels. Other infertility remedies include thyme, nutmeg, coriander, bergamot, and melissa.

How to Use Aromatherapy Remedies

Aromatherapy remedies are used by mixing them with a base oil, then rubbing them into the skin. Before applying an oil, it's a good idea to do a skin test, according to Daniele Ryman, author of *Aromatherapy: The Complete Guide to Plant and Flower Essences for Health and Beauty.* Ryman suggests putting a single drop on the skin, covering the area with a Band-Aid for 24 hours, and then inspecting it to make sure there's no redness or other reaction.

Next, you'll need a base oil to dilute your chosen remedy. Ryman advises mixing 2 to 3 drops of essential oil in a teaspoon of base oil for use on the body and 1 drop of essential oil in a teaspoon of base oil for the face. Almond and olive oil are commonly used as base oils. Other options include castor oil, grapeseed oil, soy oil, and wheat germ oil. All oils should be pure and, if possible, cold-pressed.

Once the remedy is prepared, it can be massaged into the back, chest, stomach, arms, legs, feet, or face. You can do this yourself or have your partner rub the oil into your skin. Susan Lange, O.M.D., L.Ac., co-director of the Meridian Center in Santa Monica, California, points out that the oils can be applied to certain pressure points associated with the ovaries and uterus. One point is four fingers above the tip of the ankle. Another is four fingers up from the inside of the knee joint.

Essential oils can also be used in sitz baths or breathed through a diffusor (available at some pharmacies). They should not be breathed for more than 20 minutes a day, should not be used undiluted, and should never be ingested.

Should You See a Professional?

Aromatherapy can generally be used safely at home. Keep in mind, however, that the oils are derived from the most potent part of plants and should not be overapplied. "Remember that less is more when it comes to aromatherapy," advises Mindy Green and Kathy Keville, co-authors of *Aromatherapy: A Complete Guide to the Healing Art*. "Consistent low doses are safest and most effective." Dr. Lange notes that aromatherapy can cause a detox reaction in people who haven't already worked to improve their digestion and elimination.

Ryman counsels pregnant women to avoid essential oils. She points out that many women's skin and sense of smell become more sensitive during pregnancy. Ryman also notes that certain oils can actually cause miscarriage.

The decision to treat yourself or seek professional help is an individual one, says Dr. Lange. "Some people are very good at doing self-care and are intuitive. Others need a bit of coaching to get them on track, and I will teach them how to use them. Other people really need the hand-holding and want the consultation."

To find out where to purchase aromatherapy remedies, see the Resources section.

Flower Remedies

Another member of the herbal medicine family is flower remedies. Though not as widely known as aromatherapy, this method of alternative healing can offer profound benefits for patients who seek it out.

Developed in the 1930s by British doctor Edward Bach, flower remedies are used to treat emotional imbalances that often contribute to physical illness. Bach discovered 38 plants that, when administered in certain preparations, contain potent healing properties. These preparations come in liquid form and are taken orally or applied topically.

Steven Stiteler, L.Ac., O.M.D., N.D., D.H.O.M., of Santa Monica, California, uses flower remedies to treat patients with a variety of conditions, including infertility. He says that flower remedies can counteract the body's reaction to negative emotions. "For every feeling you have, you create a corresponding neuropeptide, a small chemical messenger," explains Dr. Stiteler. "These flood the receptor sites on the cell membranes and then they influence the specific metabolism of the cells. If you have anger, you create anger neuropeptides. Joy creates joy neuropeptides; fear creates fear neuropeptides. Each one alters the metabolism. Flower remedies help to balance the neuropeptide flood."

They do this, he says, by "neutralizing the trigger" so that the body is no longer producing negative neuropeptides. "They bring you back to a still point, a state of neutrality."

By helping to restore emotional health, flower remedies can provide an important boost to physical healing. For this reason, they are often used together with other therapeutic approaches, such as acupuncture and chiropractic. Flower remedies are also prescribed by some psychiatrists as primary or accompanying treatments for a variety of psychological ailments.

Diagnosis

Whether self-prescribed or recommended by a practitioner, flower remedies are chosen based on emotional symptoms. For example, wild rose is one remedy typically prescribed for people experiencing apathy and resignation, while those plagued by suspicion and jealousy are generally given holly. Since it's common to have a range of emotional symptoms, several flower remedies are often combined into one preparation.

In addition to a thorough interview, Dr. Stiteler uses red blood cell analysis to diagnose a patient's condition. "There are certain patterns that will tell if a person is in a high state of emotional stress." He looks for certain blood chemistry patterns, such as elevated potassium, elevated glucose, reduced uric acid, and reduced magnesium. Dr. Stiteler also uses kinesiology, a form of energy medicine, to determine if the emotional stress is the result of a recent event or a deeper psychological condition.

Emotional stress can be a significant factor for women experiencing infertility. "Anger and frustration affect primarily the liver, and the liver is responsible for the conjugation of hormones, breaking them down so they can be recycled," says Dr. Stiteler. "If you're in a state of constant anxiety or fear, you can impact the adrenals, which are secondary organs in producing progesterone and estrogen."

Flower Remedies for Infertility

Many of the 38 flower remedies identified by Dr. Bach can be helpful in addressing emotional imbalances that may contribute to infertility. Dr. Stiteler has found the following ones to be particularly useful:

Heather   "This is for people who are fearful, and as a result they possess, dominate, and intervene in people's lives for the purpose of maintaining control," says Dr. Stiteler. "It's truly a remedy for insecurity." He notes that such emotions can affect the stomach and intestines, which in turn can impact the vaginal tract, making it too acidic for sperm.

Holly   Dr. Stiteler uses holly for patients who experience a lot of resentment, anger, bitterness, and jealousy. By treating these emotions, he says, women can often improve associated liver-related conditions that affect the ovaries and uterus.

Gorse   This remedy can help people whose low self-esteem results in depression and fear. These emotions, says Dr. Stiteler, can increase insulin output and are also pro-inflammatory, sometimes leading to excessive bleeding. These conditions can impair fertility.

Mustard   Unexplained depression often responds to mustard, according to Dr. Stiteler. Use of this remedy can help address related thyroid problems, often a contributing factor to infertility.

Cherry Plum   People suffering from general fear can benefit from cherry plum, says Dr. Stiteler. Alleviating fear can improve adrenal function, which plays a key role in reproductive hormonal balance.

After selecting one or more remedies, Dr. Stiteler uses red blood cell tests to check the results. "I'll administer the flowers and recheck the blood. You can see the change. We can see it balance."

Dr. Susan Lange says that although flower remedies will not

directly result in pregnancy, they "can help prompt the flow of healing." She frequently uses the Bach remedies star of Bethlehem and walnut. Star of Bethlehem is for women who experienced trauma during previous childbirth, while walnut can help overcome resistance rooted in previous abortions or miscarriages. In addition, Dr. Lange recommends the Chinese flower remedy peone, which she says can help stimulate the kind of "luscious, sensuous energy" that enhances fertility.

Dr. Lange also uses California flower remedies, available through a company called Flower Essence Services (see Resources). She recommends the following California flowers:

Mariposa Lilies This remedy improves the receptivity of the womb by helping a woman heal her own birth trauma.

Bleeding Heart Dr. Lange says that bleeding heart can clear out hidden emotions regarding a previous miscarriage or abortion. "If there is pain or guilt around abortion, the woman can actually shut down emotionally and physically. It's like their bodies are not willing to go through this again."

Black-Eyed Susan This is another remedy to help resolve a woman's birth issues. "I might use it if the difficulties of getting pregnant or carrying a child just seem too overwhelming or painful to deal with," explains Dr. Lange.

Pitcher Plant This remedy is used to strengthen physical energy in women lacking what Dr. Lange calls the "animal magnetism that is very fertile or fecund."

Golden Eardrops Dr. Lange recommends golden eardrops to help release repressed feelings from childhood that may be creating ambivalence about motherhood.

Goldenrod This remedy fosters a sense of identity separate from one's parents. "If the mother has a lot of fears, that gets projected onto the daughter, and if the daughter carries those fears, pregnancy can be very difficult," says Dr. Lange.

Sticky Monkey Flower This remedy enhances warmth and

connection, particularly for women experiencing confusion about sexuality and intimacy.

Pomegranate Women trying to balance career and family may be helped by pomegranate, which is also effective for reproductive disturbances.

Manzanita and Mugwort These remedies can ease what Dr. Lange calls the "stepdown process"—a baby's transition from the spiritual to the physical plane. "It can be quite shocking for the being. This softens and helps the preparation process."

Shooting Star and Sweet Pea Both of these remedies help prepare the womb and make it a welcoming environment.

How to Use Flower Remedies

Flower remedies are prepared in one of two ways. The first method involves placing the flowers in distilled water for several hours, then preserving the water in brandy. Certain remedies are prepared by boiling the flowers, along with their twigs and leaves, for an hour, letting the water cool, and once again preserving it in brandy.

Flower remedies can be purchased at health-food stores or through private companies (see Resources). Generally, the flower essence is mixed with purified water and a preservative such as brandy or apple cider vinegar. For mixing proportions, follow the instructions on the formula you buy. The suggested dose is four drops under the tongue, four times a day.

SUCCESS STORIES

Dr. Stiteler has found that flower remedies often work best with women who have suffered a powerful emotional trauma related to their sexuality. He recalls a patient who had been raped and sodomized as a young girl. "Ever since, she had had vaginal inflammations. Upon examining her, I found bitterness, anger, and hatred." He prescribed holly and a homeopathic remedy called *Staphysagria*. "She began to see her PMS and inflammation disappear, her menses regulate, and she started getting along better with her husband. Within 3 or 4 months, she conceived."

Should You See a Professional?

Flower remedies can be used safely and effectively at home. However, consultation with a practitioner may be helpful in monitoring your response to various remedies and coming up with the most effective combinations.

Acupuncture

Once regarded with suspicion in the West, acupuncture has now become commonplace in the United States and Europe. This deceptively complex form of medicine is used as a primary treatment for as much as 25% of the world's population.

Acupuncture was first developed in China more than 5000 years ago. It's based on the principle of chi, or energy, which circulates between organs along internal routes called meridians. By inserting very thin needles into the skin, energy flow is increased or balanced, helping to restore health. There are over 1000 acupuncture points on the body corresponding to different organs.

Diagnosis

When seeing a new patient, an acupuncturist will use a variety of methods to determine the source of the problem. In addition to asking questions, practitioners base their diagnosis on such factors as appearance, natural smell, and color. They will also take numerous pulse readings to pinpoint the source of the imbalance.

Roger Hirsh, O.M.D., L.Ac., of Beverly Hills, California, specializes in the treatment of infertility. When diagnosing a patient, he takes an extensive inventory of the woman's menstrual health.

"I ask how long their cycle is, about blood flow during menses, cramping, the color of the blood, if there's any clotting, the color of the clots, the size of the clots," says Dr. Hirsh. "We ask them if there's any pain during menstruation, if there's any relief of pain once they start, if there's pain or midcycle bleeding, vaginal fluid, if a woman is lubricated during her ovulation period. I also ask whether a woman can orgasm, whether or not there's pain with intercourse, if she's satisfied with her sensuality and sexuality."

Dr. Hirsh checks various pulse rates in different locations on the body. For instance, since kidney chi is considered vital to fertility in traditional Chinese medicine, he'll often take a woman's pulse at acupuncture point kidney 3. He palpates as many as 20 points on the abdomen, looking for tightness, tenderness, or flaccidity, and feels the spine. In addition, he observes everything from body structure to complexion and skin color to the sound of a patient's voice. "You can't hang the diagnosis on one symptom or reflex," says Dr. Hirsh. "You have to look at the big picture of the person."

Acupuncture for Infertility

Acupuncture has long been used, often together with herbal remedies, dietary changes, and mind/body exercises, to treat infertility. Dr. Daoshing Ni, L.Ac., D.O.M., Ph.D., of Santa Monica, California, says that acupuncture has been shown to be effective for a wide range of infertility-related conditions, including endometriosis, luteal-phase defect, irregular ovulation, pituitary imbalances, hyperprolactinemia, hypothyroidism, recurrent spontaneous abortion, and unexplained infertility.

PREMENSTRUAL SYNDROME

PMS symptoms are often a warning sign that a woman's menstrual system is not working as it should. According to Dr. Hirsh, PMS is usually tied to liver chi stagnation—a blockage of energy flow to the liver. "If the liver chi isn't coursing through the body correctly, the blood flow to the pelvic cavity isn't running," he explains. "The uterus and factors of the fallopian tubes are dependent upon blood innervation, and when the chi is stagnated, the blood doesn't move right. And if the liver chi is really stagnated, then you get stuck blood and endometriosis." To treat PMS-related liver chi stagnation, Dr. Hirsh stimulates liver, gallbladder, and spleen acupuncture points, in addition to using herbs, nutritional therapy, and massage.

ENDOMETRIOSIS

In traditional Chinese medicine, endometriosis is usually regarded as the result of a liver system imbalance, says Dr. Ni. "Liver system imbalance is very related to immunity and neurological systems," he explains. "We consider endometriosis an immunological, neurological condition, not just reproductive, though the disease proliferation is all in the reproductive system."

According to Dr. Ni, endometriosis is classified into four subgroups: chi stasis/blood stagnation, kidney deficiency/blood stagnation, heat stasis/blood stagnation, and cold stasis/blood stagnation. Chi stasis endometriosis, for example, will produce breast distending pain, bloating pain, dark menstrual flow with heavy clotting, and tissue discharge. "We want to release that stagnation, to circulate the chi." To do so, Dr. Ni will stimulate liver, spleen, stomach, kidney, and gallbladder acupuncture points, among others. He uses herbal remedies in conjunction with the acupuncture treatments.

HORMONAL IMBALANCE

This condition is typically traced to liver chi stagnation, kidney deficiency, and constitutional weakness, says Dr. Hirsh. Treatment focuses on liver and kidney acupuncture points.

ADRENAL DISORDERS

Dr. Hirsh says adrenal deficiency is usually produced by overwork and poor diet, along with constitutional weakness. He uses acupuncture treatments that tonify the kidney.

THYROID DISORDERS

Women with low thyroid function generally are chi deficient, according to Dr. Hirsh. He focuses on tonifying the thyroid chi. He may also work on the kidney meridians.

POLYCYSTIC OVARY SYNDROME

Although difficult to treat, polycystic ovary syndrome can respond to acupuncture. According to Dr. Hirsh, the key is to clear the body of phlegm. Primary acupuncture points include the kidney, liver, spleen, and pancreas.

COLD UTERUS

Insufficient blood supply creates a "cold" uterus in traditional Chinese medicine. It is associated with miscarriage and inability to conceive, according to Dr. Hirsh. He targets acupuncture points that increase the blood flow to the uterine cavity.

DEPRESSION

Emotional distress attributed to PMS is often brought on by liver chi stagnation, says Dr. Hirsh. "She may not have physical pain, but she may have physical mood changes and harbor qualities of anger and resentment." He treats this type of depression by using acupuncture points that work on the psyche.

SUCCESS STORIES

Dr. Y. C. Chiang treated a 41-year-old woman who had had two unsuccessful in vitro procedures. Her period was irregular, sometimes arriving early, other times late, and she had spotting for several days. She also suffered from vaginitis accompanied by itchiness and pain in the vagina and a white discharge with odor. In addition, she was experiencing dizziness and insomnia. Dr. Chiang diagnosed her with chi and blood deficiency, poor uterus function, and vaginal infection. He used acupuncture treatments to increase circulation to the meridians and the uterus, along with herbs to increase chi and blood and eliminate the infection. After 4 months, the woman became pregnant and went on to have a healthy boy.

A woman who had been diagnosed with hypothalamic amenorrhea came to see Dr. Ni. She had already tried conventional infertility treatment, which involved hormone therapy that induced ovulation but did not lead to pregnancy. By the time the woman arrived at Dr. Ni's office, "I had come to understand that I needed to treat my whole self in order to overcome this continuing health problem." After an initial interview and assessment, she began weekly acupuncture sessions. This was supplemented by an herbal tea mixture consumed three times a day. "Everything about the Chinese medicine practices and technology made me feel better, not worse. I was put in touch with the integrity of my total mind/body/energy system. I experienced a wonderful new level of health and balance. The acupuncture and herbs gave me the strength, clarity, and focus to do the work required in all aspects of myself in order to achieve healing." Five months into her work with Dr. Ni, the woman became pregnant and went on to deliver a healthy boy.

Another patient of Dr. Ni's had gone through 4 years of conventional infertility treatment, including 10 cycles of clomiphene (Clomid, which induces ovulation), a laparoscopy, two intrauterine inseminations, and a 6-month course of leuprolide (Lupron, which is used to treat endometriosis). She conceived three times, but each pregnancy ended in miscarriage. "My body was tired and my emotions spent. I also felt torn apart because I still had a deep-seated belief that I could have a baby." Originally, the woman intended to use acupuncture and herbs to strengthen her body while continuing with standard infertility treatment. Dr. Ni suggested that she try his program alone for a few months. Three months later, she conceived, and this time successfully held the pregnancy.

Should You See a Professional?

Acupuncture should be administered only by a trained professional. There are thousands of licensed acupuncturists in North America, including a growing number of medical doctors who also perform acupuncture.

Homeopathy

Developed 200 years ago by Samuel Hahnemann, classical homeopathy is a natural form of medicine in which extremely dilute preparations of plants, animals, and minerals are given to patients according to the law of similars. This law states that it's possible to cure a sick person of a symptom with a remedy that would cause that same symptom in a healthy person.

Classical homeopathy embraces a holistic approach to healing, incorporating dietary changes, supplementation, exercise, and mind/body techniques. Acupuncture and some herbal medicines can interfere with homeopathic remedies, however, and some practitioners advise patients not to use these therapies while using homeopathic preparations. Homeopathic remedies are labeled with a number and a letter, indicating how many times they've been shaken and diluted.

Diagnosis

The homeopathic diagnosis consists almost entirely of an interview with the patient that may last from 45 to 120 minutes. The selection of a remedy is dependent on the patient's story and how she tells it.

For women experiencing fertility problems, homeopathy is most often used with a more general view of the woman and her menstrual situation. A patient will be asked to describe everything about her chief complaints, from menstrual symptoms to the way she feels about her period. The practitioner will try to find out as much as possible about a patient before considering possible remedies.

Homeopathic Remedies for Infertility

Here's an example of how a woman's entire profile—physical, emotional, and psychological—is used to determine a homeopathic remedy. A patient has been grieving ever since her mother died and can't get pregnant. There are half a dozen remedies for someone who is grieving, is unable to conceive, and whose mother has died. Therefore, the homeopath will also take into consideration body type and character. For example, a woman who is thin, lithe, and irritable would receive a different prescription than one who is mellow, slow, slightly anxious, and conscientious.

Homeopathy works hand in hand with common-sense practical advice. For instance, if a woman is a marathon runner, thin to the point of having scanty periods, and has lost some of her sex drive, a practitioner would likely prescribe *Sepia* and would suggest that the patient does less running so that she improves her chances of having normal periods.

Another remedy to consider for infertility is *Natrum muri-*

aticum, which is derived from sea salt. *Natrum* is typically given to women who tend to be serious and refined, reserved about their emotions in general and grief in particular. They may have associated problems of migraines (extending back to childhood), cold sores, and a tendency to depression. They often started menstruating at a late age and may skip periods in times of grief.

Coffea, in contrast, is used to treat infertility in women who are lively and excitable. Such patients can develop an aversion to sex because everything feels too sensitive, including their vagina, which can't bear the intensity of intercourse. Within a month or two, *Coffea*—also commonly prescribed for insomnia—should bring about improvement in some complaints. If a woman first starts sleeping through the night and a month later can have sex without feeling too uncomfortable, the remedy is probably working and should be continued for several months to see if conception occurs. (Homeopathic remedies for infertility are generally taken for a minimum of 3 months, and sometimes for several years.)

Nux vomica can enhance the fertility of the workaholic personality, says Katherine Zieman, N.D, L.M., an associate professor of obstetrics and fertility at the National College of Naturopathic Medicine in Portland, Oregon. These women typically have a bad diet, poor digestion, inadequate sleep, and tend to drink a lot of coffee to keep themselves going. Their ovulation pattern may be off because of fatigue, which may also have caused them to miss a couple of periods. "*Nux vomica* is for people who are working way too hard, to the point where it's breaking them down and they crave stimulants to keep them going," says Dr. Zieman. "It will help them get off the hamster wheel." In addition to homeopathy, she'll recommend dietary changes, nutritional supplementation, herbs, and lifestyle modification.

Pulsatilla is another remedy that can be useful for infertility.

According to Dr. Zieman, it is prescribed for women with soft, yielding personalities who need a lot of affection. They often have heavy periods, experience difficulty processing fats, and are overweight.

SUCCESS STORIES

A 36-year-old woman came to see co-author Dr. Deborah Gordon after having repeated miscarriages. As homeopathy texts list at least 126 possible remedies for miscarriage, Dr. Gordon asked some specific questions about the patient's menstrual history. She found out that the woman had cysts on her ovaries and a uterine fibroid, she sometimes spotted between periods or after intercourse, and her periods had gotten shorter. Speaking more about her general health, the patient complained of pain in the knees, which kept her from competing in tennis as aggressively as she wanted. Her schedule didn't allow much time for recreation anyway, as she was a perfectionist and kept busy remodeling a bed-and-breakfast with her husband as well as caring for two growing children. Dr. Gordon also found out that the patient had had a problem with asthma and constipation when she was young, and that there was skin cancer in her family. Ultimately, all this information led to the choice of *Carcinosin*. The woman conceived within 6 to 12 months of starting the remedy and gave birth to a healthy boy.

"If you look at the broad symptom of tendency to abortion, this remedy is not one of the ones normally chosen," says Dr. Gordon. "It's not even used for sterility. But it was the right one. She might have given herself a different remedy that probably wouldn't have worked, but a lengthy interview which took into account the whole person led to the selection of the right remedy."

In another case, an overweight, hardworking, 26-year-old

mother of one came to see Dr. Gordon for the dual complaints of exhaustion and inability to conceive. She had a 2-year-old, was working nearly full-time, and was the primary home-maker, as her husband worked more than full-time. She had been unable to exercise, which she never enjoyed anyway, and had gained about 20 pounds. Her periods had become quite heavy and painful. These symptoms clearly called for *Calcarea carbonica*. "The prescription resulted in normalizing of her period, the ability to decide to cut back enough on work so she wasn't exhausted, a mild exercise program to reinvigorate her—and a nice baby girl about 6 months later," says Dr. Gordon.

Should You See a Professional?

Self-prescribing is possible, but if it's not effective, the objec-tivity and experience of a professional can make a difference. If you choose a remedy and haven't achieved conception in 3 months, a professional homeopath should be consulted.

CHAPTER EIGHT

Exercise, Movement Therapy, and Massage

At the heart of the Six-Step Natural Fertility Program is the relationship each woman has with her body. There is no better way to nurture that relationship than through a regular, moderate exercise routine.

Over the past few decades, as medical science has discovered the far-ranging health benefits of physical fitness, more and more people have started to get in shape. Exercise regimens run the gamut from old-fashioned activities such as running, swimming, and dancing to such new sensations as power walking, spinning, and Tae-Bo.

Anyone who has made the transition from couch potato to fitness enthusiast knows just how strong the healing powers of movement can be. And scientific research has now confirmed what our bodies have been telling us all along, documenting the positive effects exercise has on cardiovascular function, the immune system, bone density and integrity, sleep, emotional well-being, and myriad other aspects of human health.

For women trying to get pregnant, exercise can play a vital role. On a physical level, fitness routines can help strengthen the reproductive organs, increase circulation to the pelvis, and balance the hormones. "You want to get on a good exercise program before you get pregnant," says Cynthia Watson, M.D., of Santa Monica, California. "When you're exercising regularly, you are increasing the oxygen-carrying capacity of cells and muscles."

Exercise also offers important psychological benefits, providing an outlet for the anxiety that often goes hand in hand with efforts to conceive. "There's something about the infertility process that, on a stress level, is unlike anything else people face, individually for the woman and mutually for the couple," observes Sat Jivan Kaur Khalsa, a New York City–based kundalini yoga instructor who has worked with many women trying to get pregnant. "Kundalini yoga can help people who are actively involved in that process. I have found it very helpful just to de-stress and get through the day-to-day grind."

In this chapter, we'll look at movement therapies such as yoga, chi gung, and tai chi that have long been used to enhance fertility. We'll also discuss the healing properties of massage, both as a way to promote relaxation and to increase intimacy in your relationship. In addition, we'll review other techniques such as chiropractic and myofascial therapy that can help prepare your body for pregnancy.

Everything in Moderation

As with eating, people tend to fall on one side or the other of the fitness spectrum. Far too many people lead sedentary lifestyles that consist mainly of sitting in an office during the day and sitting in front of the TV or computer at night. On the other extreme are those who seem to live at the gym, pushing their bodies to the limits of endurance.

In preparing for pregnancy, the best approach to exercise is moderation. That means creating a workout routine that keeps you active but doesn't put too much of a strain on your body.

For women who are experiencing menstrual and ovulatory irregularities that may be tied to excessive weight, exercise is a critical part of restoring healthy reproductive function. A regular fitness routine not only will help take off pounds but will improve circulation, reduce stress, and stimulate immune function.

Don't go overboard, however. "It's important that it not be so strenuous that it stops you from ovulating," says Katherine Zieman, N.D., L.M., of Portland, Oregon. "It all comes back to stress. If you're too stressed, you won't ovulate. The body doesn't understand the difference between the stress of work or of a famine or of being on a forced march."

The main danger of overexertion is reduced body fat. Women whose body fat falls below a certain level can have difficulty getting pregnant, since adequate fat is needed for normal menstrual function. This is why professional female athletes often have irregular periods.

Christiane Northrup, M.D., notes that amenorrhea is more common in young, childless women athletes than in those who have had children. "After a woman has had children, she is less likely to develop this problem because childbearing appears to make her hormonal system difficult to suppress via extreme exercise," writes Dr. Northrup in her book *Women's Bodies, Women's Wisdom.* She notes that poor diet is a key factor in menstrual irregularities among female athletes, since the combination of excessive exercise and insufficient nutrition increases the chance of cycle disturbances.

Yoga

Developed thousands of years ago, yoga is a complex system of healing used by tens of millions of people. Although it originated in the East, it has now become popular throughout the Western world.

There are numerous kinds of yoga, but all involve the integration of three basic elements: postures, breath, and meditation. The combination of these practices can have profound health benefits, helping ease everything from hypertension to arthritis to insomnia.

Yoga has traditionally been used for a variety of menstrual problems, including premenstrual syndrome (PMS) and menopausal symptoms. Since the 1980s, more and more women have begun practicing yoga both before and during pregnancy, while leading medical institutions such as Harvard University have incorporated it into their infertility programs.

While yoga classes are easy to find in most cities, certain instructors have more experience working with women and reproduction. Here are the approaches of three leading teachers in the field of yoga and fertility.

Margie Canty and Hatha Yoga

Margie Canty, R.N., of Boston, Massachusetts, knows how disconnected women can become from their bodies. And she knows how powerful a tool yoga can be to restore that connection.

Canty, who has been teaching yoga for 20 years, is coordinator of the hatha yoga/body awareness component of Beth Israel Deaconess Hospital's mind/body program. She works with patients facing a range of conditions, including infertility, showing them yoga techniques that can help improve their physical and emotional health.

In Canty's infertility classes, women learn gentle yoga movements drawn primarily from the hatha school, the most widely used yoga practice. Some of the exercises promote overall relaxation, whereas others specifically stimulate the pelvic organs. For example, Canty cites a pose where a woman brings the knee up to the chest while lying in a supine position and breathing. The idea is to soften the belly and stretch the lower back, which has a relaxing effect on the pelvis while stimulating the digestion and elimination organs.

"There are poses that are known to stimulate and relax the reproductive organs, that bring blood flow to the pelvis," says Canty. "When people are stressed, one of the physiological effects is that the blood flow is shunted away to the muscles. The exercises that facilitate relaxation bring that blood flow back."

Yoga's ability to relax the body can have a profound effect on a woman's ability to conceive, says Canty. "We can be in fight-and-flight response or in feed-and-breed response, where we can be more open to being pregnant or even being sexual. . . . The relaxation response is a way of moving more into that kind of physiology where the body is feeding itself the chemicals that facilitate pregnancy."

While Canty teaches women numerous yoga poses for general and reproductive health, her approach goes beyond mere exercises. Through yoga, she helps women change their perceptions of their bodies. "The main thing that I stress is the concept of redeveloping the relationship with the body," states Canty. "That means letting go of seeing the body as utilitarian, and seeing it more as something one would want to develop a relationship with, the same as you would want to develop a relationship with anyone in your life."

Canty outlines three principles that form the basis of her program. The first is body awareness. "We encourage people to start paying attention to the body in a respectful way," she explains. "Part of that is just simple awareness. You bring your body to physical awareness in hatha, and hopefully that will proliferate throughout the day." The key here is focusing on the breath, which Canty notes often reflects a person's emotional state. "If we're stressed, the breath is shallow. If we're relaxed, it's deep and open." By getting patients to regulate their breath, she says, "we help people to slow down and feel what is happening in the body and pay attention to it in a respectful way."

The second principle is language. "We want to help patients start knowing what their inner physical sensations are so they can respond compassionately," states Canty. Although this may sound easy, she says, it's not, because so many people have lost touch with their body's basic needs.

"I like to talk about the body being an innocent animal whose only purpose is to sustain our life. It's constantly giving us messages to proceed throughout the day in a way that's most healthy to us. But we have this wonderful cerebral cortex getting so much information, and we're usually in the higher reaches of the brain. We have to learn to drop down and hear the most primitive types of messages—we're thirsty; we need to rest. There are so many things we do because we haven't slowed down and paid attention to what's really going on."

The final principle is letting go of judgment. "When you're with the people you love and care about the most, they're not judging you, you can be yourself," says Canty. "That's the attitude you want to develop with your body, to let go of judgment."

In addition to teaching women directly in a group setting, Canty provides participants with tapes they can use at home to guide them through various poses. This is an important part of the program, because it helps the women achieve a sense of self-efficacy, says Canty. "They can practice hatha yoga for a half-hour and then be in a very different place. That's a very empowering tool, that they can change their internal environment without taking a drug, without being dependent on someone or something to do that."

Judith Lasater and Restorative Yoga

Based in the San Francisco Bay Area, Judith Lasater, Ph.D., P.T., has been teaching yoga since 1971. An internationally respected educator, she has written extensively about the therapeutic benefits of yoga.

Over the years, Dr. Lasater has worked with many women before and during pregnancy. Like Margie Canty, she takes a holistic view of her students. "I approach the woman like any student who walks through the door—how can I support this person in their life right now, help them become whole and healthy in their life, which may or may not include getting pregnant," says Dr. Lasater.

Much of her instruction is devoted to what she calls restorative yoga. Based largely on the teachings of Indian yoga master B. K. S. Iyengar, this approach emphasizes poses that promote "active relaxation." The idea, explains Dr. Lasater, is to restore health by reducing stress. "In general, restorative poses are for those times when you feel weak, fatigued, or stressed from your daily activities," she writes, noting that these poses are particularly helpful before, during, or after major life events.

Among the exercises Dr. Lasater teaches are inverted poses, in which the uterus is higher than the heart and the effects of gravity are reversed. She notes that scientific research has found that these poses have a dramatic impact on hormone levels.

To enhance fertility, Dr. Lasater focuses on the prana, or energy, called apana. Centered in the abdomen, apana is feminine energy. "We want to do things that stimulate apana," she says. "We want to increase the energy and make sure it is really good in the belly and the endocrine system as a whole."

Some of the exercises recommended by Dr. Lasater, such as the supported bridge and elevated legs-up-the-wall poses, are designed primarily to put the body in the relaxed state known as the parasympathetic mode. "These are very cooling and quieting to the brain," says Dr. Lasater. "Our culture tends to be in sympathetic nervous mode. When you're doing that, your body is either going to be eaten by the tiger or eat the tiger. It doesn't need to repair, digest, eliminate, and reproduce. Those are long-term activities. It needs to run or fight."

Other exercises target specific areas of the body. The supported crossed-leg pose, for example, cools and relaxes the reproductive organs, along with the liver and kidneys. The mountain brook pose improves digestion, a key factor in optimal fertility. (*Note:* For pregnant women, all of these exercises except the supported crossed-leg pose should be avoided after the first trimester.) To help maintain or restore hormonal balance, Dr. Lasater advises creating a routine that includes more inverted poses. However, she cautions that these poses should not be practiced during your period, as they can interfere with menstrual flow.

The following poses, along with more than two dozen others, are described and illustrated in *Relax and Renew:*

SUPPORTED BRIDGE POSE

Place bolsters or several blankets on the floor. They should be 6 to 12 inches from the floor, depending on your height. Sit down, and, using your arms, stretch out slowly on your back,

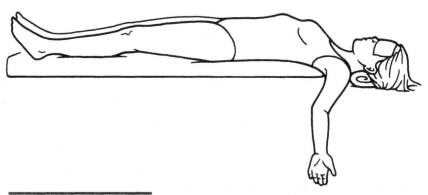

Supported bridge pose

with your head and neck below the rest of your body, supported by a rolled-up towel. Your shoulders should touch the floor. Let your arms rest off to the side, and cover your eyes with an eye bag. Dr. Lasater advises that if you feel any discomfort in the lower back, bend your knees and place your feet either on the bolsters or on the floor. Once you are in position, focus on your breathing, particularly your lungs and ribs. Continue for up to 15 minutes. Afterward, lie on the floor with your lower legs on the bolsters for a few minutes.

SUPPORTED CROSSED-LEG POSE

Sit down on the floor by the side of a chair and cross your legs at the ankle. Lean forward, folding your arms, and place them on the chair. Let your forehead rest on your arms. Dr. Lasater notes that some people may need to sit on the corner of one or more folded blankets to maintain the proper curve of the lower back. She also says that the neck should not sag when resting on the forehead; if it does, pull the chin back a little and in. If you have difficulty bending forward, you can elevate the chair with blankets or turn it so that the back faces you. Once you're in position, focus on your breathing. Do this pose for 3

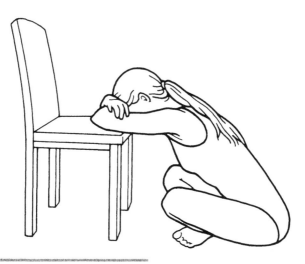

Supported crossed-legged pose

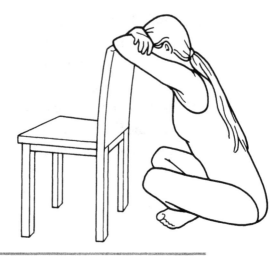

Variation for supported crossed-legged pose

minutes, then repeat with the other ankle on top. Afterward, sit up slowly and lean back on your hands.

Sat Jivan Kaur Khalsa and Kundalini Yoga

Trying to fit exercise into a hectic schedule can be a daunting task. And squeezing in a quick trip to the gym after work, although better than nothing, might do little for your physical or emotional health.

A better option may be kundalini yoga. "It's particularly applicable for people with very busy lives, and works quickly," says Sat Jivan Kaur Khalsa. As director of Kundalini Yoga East, located in New York City, she knows all about helping people incorporate yoga into life in the fast lane.

Over the past three decades, Khalsa has taught yoga to many women experiencing infertility. Her approach combines yogic meditations and poses designed to get the body's glandular system working at peak condition. "We regard glands as the guardians of health," she says. "When glands function properly, the rest of the organs function properly."

The first step, according to Khalsa, is to make sure a

woman's period is regular. Among the techniques she uses for women with menstrual problems is a meditation that works on the pituitary gland through sound and touch. The exercise involves touching the thumbs to the fingertips in a specific order while pronouncing certain words with the mouth wide open. This has an effect on the hypothalamus, which in turn affects the pituitary. "The hypothalamus and pituitary can be stimulated and helped to synchronize through the rhythmic pulsation of sound and breath," says Khalsa, adding that eye focus is also helpful, as it works on the pituitary as well. She reports that this meditation has been very successful for women with amenorrhea.

Khalsa uses numerous poses to revitalize the reproductive organs. One, called the half-wheel pose, can be done in bed. "Lying on your back, you bring your feet up near the buttocks, reach down to your ankles, and lift the pelvis as high as you can. This stretches the thigh very directly. Within 5 to 10 lifts, you will start to feel the connection from the knee to the top of the thigh to the ovary. Then exhale and roll the spine down." By doing 15 to 30 repetitions, says Khalsa, you stimulate the meridian, or energy corridor, that runs through the ovaries, helping them to relax.

A second exercise is the rock pose, which also relaxes the ovaries. It can be done on both sides of the body. On the left side, it targets the stomach, heart, kidney, spleen, and adrenal gland. On the right side, it stimulates the gallbladder, kidney, thyroid, and adrenal gland. This pose is best learned with the help of an instructor.

Getting Started

Although it's possible to learn yoga from books and videos, you'll probably pick it up faster and get more satisfaction by taking a class with a trained teacher. Margie Canty advises women to look for an instructor who pays attention not only to technique but to process and relaxation. "Focusing just on technique might set up another perfectionistic chore to do," observes Canty. "The best kind of teacher is someone who helps people to relax and establish a sense of self-efficacy by being able to use these postures to bring about relaxation in their life, not to become the yoga icon."

It's also extremely important to remember that some yoga poses that can enhance fertility should not be done during pregnancy. If you have any doubts, consult with both your health care practitioner and your yoga instructor.

Chi Gung and Tai Chi

Like yoga, chi gung is an ancient system of natural healing that uses energy flow to maintain and restore health. Developed in China, where it remains a fixture of everyday life, chi gung has become a popular practice in the West.

Chi gung works on the principle of chi, or energy, either moving chi (energy) that is stuck or building up chi if it's deficient, explains Roger Jahnke, O.M.D., director of Health Action in Santa Barbara, California, and chairperson of the National Qi Gong Association. This is done by combining three elements: movement, breath, and mental focus. In chi gung, a person gently moves the body and adjusts the posture, deepens and lengthens the breath, and clears the mind. Regular practice, says Dr. Jahnke, can improve immune response, increase resistance to disease, lower heart rate and blood pressure, and yield a wealth of other benefits.

Tai chi, a form of chi gung, produces similar results. However, it takes longer to learn, and thus is less practical unless you can devote a significant amount of time to practice.

Chi gung has a long history in helping women prepare for pregnancy. "Chi gung is the Lamaze method from thousands of years ago," says Dr. Jahnke. "All of the best wisdom brought to bear on the whole self-care side of birth and pregnancy that we called Lamaze was really developed by traditional culture."

By reducing stress, chi gung can be an important component of a natural approach to conception. "In fertility, one thing that is a part of the problem in many cases is a low level of sustained inner tension," observes Dr. Jahnke, who has worked with many women trying to get pregnant. "Chi gung, because it is focused on relaxation as a method for balancing energy, is an immensely powerful tool in both normal pregnancy and fertility."

Chi gung, explains Dr. Jahnke, moves the nervous system out of the "doing" state and into the "rest-and-repair" state. This transition is characterized by a change in the mix of neurotransmitters, which carry messages from the brain to the rest of the body. "Because of the shift in neurotransmitters, there's a whole cascade of neurological and hormonal effects that can arise, many of which capacitate or optimize conception," says Dr. Jahnke.

Chi gung can have a positive impact on fertility in other ways as well. It increases delivery of oxygen and nutrition to the glands, the organs, the cells, and the brain. Chi gung also stimulates the lymph system, the body's primary detoxification system, helping to improve elimination. In addition, it has a toning effect on the body, including the reproductive organs. All of these factors contribute to optimal fertility.

Y. C. Chiang, O.M.D., Ph.D., of El Cerrito, California, has treated hundreds of women with infertility over several decades, and says that chi gung and tai chi can be very helpful for patients without any serious structural impairment of the reproductive system. "These exercises change the nature and imbalances of the body and achieve balance of the chi and blood," states Dr. Chiang. "Infertility is due to imbalance of the chi and blood. When chi and blood become irregular, then the biological functions of the body become irregular. Tai chi and chi gung are effective because these exercises increase . . . blood and chi circulation."

According to Dr. Jahnke, there are two ways to approach chi gung. The first is to devote a certain amount of time each day to practicing chi gung breathing and movement exercises. The other is to strive to be in a chi gung state throughout the course of the day using a Chinese concept called mind intent. "That means no matter what you're doing, you remain in the low-grade practice of chi gung all the time," explains Dr. Jahnke. "Sustaining [good] body posture, moving it gently, focusing on deepening and lengthening the breath, and calming the nervous system by clearing the mind—these are things people can do anywhere." No matter what you're doing—shopping, eating, driving—you can apply the principles of chi gung. "It's more than just a technique," he says. "It really is a way of being."

Of course, you don't have to make chi gung a way of life to benefit from it. Dr. Jahnke recommends a daily routine of 20 to 40 minutes, while encouraging people to apply the techniques as much as possible during the rest of the day.

Daoshing Ni, L.Ac., D.O.M., Ph.D., of Santa Monica, California, says that chi gung can be customized to work on a particular organ or system. The exercises are performed much like yoga postures and have similar benefits. The crane head and dragon head movements both strengthen the kidney system, which according to traditional Chinese medicine correlates to reproductive essence. The crane skimming and dotting the water exercise focuses on the liver system and is helpful for women who have chi stagnation manifesting in such conditions as endometriosis and PMS, both of which can contribute to infertility.

Gilles Marin, director of the Chi Nei Tsang Institute in Berkeley, California, uses a number of chi gung movements that target the reproductive organs. These include contraction and relaxation of the anal and vaginal areas, as well as exercises that focus on the breath as it rises from the pelvic floor to the sacrum and then up to the shoulder blades.

Dr. Jahnke, Dr. Ni, and Marin all emphasize that chi gung works best as part of a larger program that includes such vital elements as proper diet, nutritional supplementation, and adequate sleep. Dr. Jahnke recalls the case of one patient to illustrate the role of chi gung in a comprehensive approach to enhancing fertility through natural medicine.

"The couple had had one child, but the second pregnancy was not happening. They did all the testing, and found that while some of the clinical factors were somewhat deficient, they weren't in the danger zone. Through a nice, balanced program of chi gung, dietary change, herbal formulas, and one or two acupuncture treatments, she got pregnant." The chi gung element of the program consisted of 20 to 40 minutes of focused practice a day, along with a sustained effort to apply chi gung principles on an ongoing basis.

Chi Gung in Practice: Gilles Marin and the Chi Nei Tsang Institute

As director of the Chi Nei Tsang Institute, Gilles Marin has used chi gung to help many women get pregnant. But chi gung's power, says Marin, comes not so much from the specific movements as from its ability to awaken in women a deeper, more holistic self-awareness.

Marin's approach combines breathing, standing, and movement that he says allows women to get in touch with their biological rhythms. "It helps them to feel what their needs are—eating, sleeping, relaxation."

For women trying to get pregnant, it's particularly important that they uncover any underlying issues that may be compromising their fertility, says Marin. "If there is an emotional charge in that part of the body—fear, too much anger—getting in touch with that is very important to free the space for pregnancy." Chi gung does this by increasing the flow of chi, which Marin defines as both energy and information. "Once we're able to make the chi circulate within the body, we get in touch with the information that is there."

He cites the example of women with very hectic lives who are having difficulty getting pregnant. Marin helps devise a program of chi gung and other natural therapies that allows them to get in touch with their need for more time and space. This often translates into a decision to work less hours and use the newfound free time for relaxation.

One of the most common problems Marin encounters is women who eat at irregular hours or skip meals altogether. "The body lives on the clock, on daily rhythms. If the body needs to be very hungry in order to be fed, you're sending the message that there's starvation out there. This situation is not good for procreation. The mind knows we live in abundance, but the body is hungry. We can't send double messages like that."

Another common problem is inadequate rest. Marin recalls working with several women during the same period of time who were trying to conceive. "Through doing chi gung they realized they were starving for sleep," he says, noting that chi gung helps to increase the parasympathetic response in the body, which can improve both the quality and duration of sleep.

"For me, the main reason for infertility is that the energy is not there," explains Marin. "The body doesn't have the requirements it needs to allow pregnancy to happen. Chi gung makes the connection between physical needs, mental understanding, and emotional adjustment."

Getting Started

As with yoga, you can buy tapes and books with instructions on how to do chi gung or tai chi, but you'll be better off taking a class with an experienced teacher. Once you've learned the basics, you can then devise your own routine.

In choosing between a class in tai chi or chi gung, Dr. Jahnke suggests that chi gung may be more pragmatic for most people. "If you have a lot of time to learn 108 movements, go ahead and learn tai chi. For everyone else who lives in the modern world and has to prioritize, some of the more brief forms of chi gung are easier to learn and apply."

Here are two simple chi gung practices recommended by Dr. Jahnke.

CIRCULATING CHI

Begin by rubbing your hands together. Move the palms of your hands upward across your cheeks, eyes, and forehead, then along the top and side of your head. Continue down the back of your neck and across your shoulders until you reach your shoulder joint. Proceed under the arms and the down the sides. At the lower edge of the rib cage, move your hands to your back, across the buttocks, down the back and sides of the legs, and out the sides of the feet. Continue on the inside of the feet and the inner legs, up the front of the torso, and onto the face again. Repeat.

TWISTING THE WAIST

Stand with your feet at shoulder width and twist your torso from side to side. Let your arms swing freely, and rotate your head as far as comfortably possible. Breathe deeply and relax as you move.

Massage

Everyone knows how wonderful it feels to get a massage. And for good reason: with just the touch of a hand, we can reconnect with the most fundamental part of our nature. "One of the greatest gifts of massage is that it brings people back into their bodies," says Rebecca Bowler, L.M.T. "Most people walk around not in their bodies."

The power of massage goes beyond mere tactile pleasure. Extensive research has shown that therapeutic massage can have profound healing effects. Pain reduction, increased circulation, improved elimination of toxins, and enhanced vitality are among the many benefits attributed to massage.

Massage has much to offer women trying to get pregnant. Stress reduction, perhaps the most obvious reason people seek out massage, can have a direct effect on hormonal balance and ovulation, while better circulation and elimination are both important components of optimal fertility.

Both yoga and chi gung have developed self-massage techniques to stimulate the reproductive system. Khalsa instructs her students how to do yogic self-massage to relieve stress. She recommends that before women get out of bed, they massage the ovaries with their fingertips. "People have a lot of tension in that area. If they massage it for several minutes, it will change their mood and temperament," states Khalsa, noting that such tension can suppress ovulation and even cause cystic ovaries. She also suggests massaging the breasts with the palms for further stress reduction.

According to Dr. Roger Jahnke, classical chi gung includes self-applied massage. Stimulating points on the ears, hands, and feet, along with acupuncture points throughout the body, can ease tension in the pelvic area.

Dr. Daoshing Ni uses a form of Chinese massage called tuina along with acupressure. "A lot of times this body work can stimulate a wider area in the waist, the lower back, and in turn the spinal nerves," says Dr. Ni. "This can stimulate the pelvic area, which can facilitate better circulation to the uterus and ovaries, and improve follicular genesis, follicular quality, and uterine receptivity." He notes that he'll often use massage with infertility patients who have poor circulation, chronic back and neck pain, and knee troubles.

Gilles Marin focuses on abdominal massage. "It's very important to touch the organs in this area—the liver, the stomach, the pancreas—because a lot of stagnation in the lower abdomen is coming from lack of movement," explains Marin. "This increases metabolism and revitalizes the organs."

Massage is also a tremendously effective way to build intimacy in a relationship. This is true anytime, but particularly during periods of tension or anxiety, which so often are present when a woman is trying to get pregnant.

If you think you have to be an expert to give a good massage, think again. "Massage is like 80% presence and 20% technique," says Bowler. "The whole idea is that if you can be extremely present with your partner through your touch, you don't have to know what you're doing for them to receive that and be met on a deep and spiritual level."

More important than technique is trust—an area where partners in a relationship usually have an advantage over a professional. "There's a whole art to receiving massage, and a lot of people don't have that," remarks Bowler. "What's critical to learning that is trusting the person you're letting in. If you're intimate with someone, you're already set up to receive in a really deep and loving way that can be relaxing and healing."

Also essential to a good massage is open communication. You need to let your partner know what feels good and what doesn't, where you want to be touched and where you don't. "Feedback is very important," says Bowler. "People ask me, 'How does my body feel to you?' and I say, 'How does your body feel to *you*?' I can feel knots or heat or inflammation or crunchiness and reflect that back, but the authority is the body itself."

One thing to keep in mind with massage is that deeper is not always better. "A soft, gentle touch can go a long way," says Marin. "In order to listen, the touch has to be very gentle. The approach is not to fix but to allow the person being massaged to feel themselves and to enjoy being in touch with that part of the body."

Although massage between couples is immensely satisfying, receiving a massage from a professional also has its rewards. For one, massage therapists can use their knowledge of the body to respond to specific problems. Another advantage, particularly for women, is that massage therapists are trained to separate sex from touching, allowing their clients to enjoy a sensual experience without the pressure and expectations that frequently accompany sexual intimacy.

Professional massage can also enhance couples massage. "It enables the person who's receiving to learn how they like to be touched, and they can take that into their partnership," observes Bowler.

Another skill you can pick up from a massage therapist is an understanding of how to give physical pleasure in a non-sexual way. Although massage may lead to lovemaking, it is not in itself a sexual act, and thus can be used to rebuild intimacy between people whose primary form of physical communication is sex. "It's a really loving way to communicate with somebody that you care about, to tell them that they matter to you and not just for sexual purposes," states Bowler. "The value of the sacredness and sanctity of the body takes on a whole different meaning when we can learn how to touch people without it having to lead anywhere, and that's what true intimacy is about."

Other Kinds of Body Work and Physiotherapy

There are numerous varieties of touch-based healing, from reflexology to acupressure. Many of these techniques can be used to enhance fertility.

One of the most popular forms of hands-on treatment is chiropractic. Based on the premise that the nervous system controls and coordinates all functions in the body, chiropractic care is designed to help the body self-heal and self-regulate. This is done by removing interferences caused by misalignments in the spine, which restores proper nerve flow.

Christine Anderson, D.C., D.I.C.C.P., of Los Angeles, California, specializes in pediatrics and pregnancy. She has worked with many women trying to conceive and has found chiropractic care to be helpful. She says that certain misalignments can directly affect fertility. For instance, misalignments in the first cervical vertebra can impact blood supply to the pituitary gland and potentially cause miscarriage, explains Dr. Anderson, while the seventh cervical vertebra can affect thyroid gland function and in turn disrupt ovulation.

The ninth and tenth thoracic vertebrae affect the adrenal glands, which also play a vital role in ovulation, and the twelfth thoracic vertebra can create problems with fallopian tube, ovarian, and uterine function. Misalignments in the sacral and coccygeal areas may compromise the cervix, another key factor in conception.

The cranial-sacral region is especially important for fertility, says Dr. Anderson, as it affects both the brain and cerebral spinal fluid. "If the pump is affected, toxins can build up and affect the nervous system, causing misalignments. This directly affects the pituitary gland, which is responsible for FSH and LH."

Complementary Body Work: Pluta Movement Therapeutics

Nataly Pluta, P.T., of Del Mar, California, has developed an approach to infertility that integrates several kinds of movement and touch-based therapy. Motivated by her own unhappy experience with fertility drugs, Pluta, who ultimately decided to be childless, has done research into reducing pelvic tension. She is now applying the results of her inquiry in the hopes of helping other women trying to get pregnant.

Working with both partners, Pluta begins by doing a comprehensive muscular and postural assessment. Muscular imbalances in women, she explains, can inhibit circulation, normal nervous system flow, and proper nutrient flow, all of which contribute to fertility.

Pluta's treatment program consists of three elements: yoga, Rolfing, and myofascial therapy. In the yoga component, she teaches couples restorative exercises such as the pigeon pose, the fish pose, and the corpse pose. Most of these poses are done lying on the back, with plenty of support from pillows. The goal, says Pluta, is to stretch the pelvic muscles and relax and increase circulation to the pelvic area.

Rolfing is a form of intense manual massage developed by biochemist Ida P. Rolf. Pluta focuses on the psoas muscle, located deep in the pelvis. "Tightness of the muscle inhibits autonomic nervous system flow to the ovaries and uterus," states Pluta. She also works on the piriformis muscle in the buttocks. "This releases the hips, which releases the spine and the sacrum, thereby increasing neural flow, circulation, and nutrient flow."

The third part of Pluta's program is myofascial therapy. Fascia is the thin membrane covering of muscles, nerves, and every other element of the body. According to myofascial therapy, manipulating the fascia has therapeutic benefits. Pluta uses an exercise called the leg pole release, in which the leg is pulled in different directions with constant pressure. This releases the fascia from the rib cage down, once again increasing neural and nutrient flow as well as circulation, says Pluta.

In addition to the couples sessions, Pluta conducts group workshops, which provide participants with support during what may be a difficult time in their lives. She has found that her program not only helps improve health and vitality but also can heighten intimacy by teaching couples how to perform these techniques together.

Body Wisdom

There are countless ways to integrate exercise, movement therapies, and massage into your life. The most important thing is to learn to listen to your body and then let it guide you. This can be an immensely satisfying experience, one that will not only increase your chances of getting pregnant, but will give you a greater sense of physical, emotional, and spiritual well-being.

CHAPTER NINE

Breaking the Stress Cycle— Mind/Body Remedies for Relaxation

It's well documented that physical exercise can do wonders for our emotional health. But can the mind help heal the body?

The answer is a resounding yes, as evidenced in the booming field of mind/body medicine. Through the work and writings of such notable visionaries as Norman Cousins and Deepak Chopra, the Western world has begun to understand what peoples in the East have known for centuries: that physical health cannot be separated from psychological and emotional well-being.

Before the 1980s, most doctors tended to regard health as a matter of simple biology. If anything interfered with the body's proper functioning, a drug was pulled off the shelf or a patient was referred to a surgeon.

Of course, medications and surgical procedures are essential in the treatment of certain illnesses. But there's a growing realization among health care practitioners that the mind can be a potent force as well in the healing process.

Greater appreciation of the mind/body connection comes partly through our increased participation in a global society. As the world's cultures have become more entwined, we have started to seek out the healing traditions of societies in which the interconnection between mind and body is taken for granted. For much of the world, practices such as meditation and relaxation are considered essential to basic health. This integrationist approach, once dismissed in the West, is now the focus of intense public as well as scientific interest.

The research community has put significant resources into this new frontier. Prestigious academic institutions such as Stanford University, University of Massachusetts, and Harvard University have created mind/body programs, studying every-thing from the chemistry of emotions to the effect of stress reduction on cardiovascular health. Countless studies have confirmed long-held beliefs about the relationship between physical health and such factors as stress and depression. In so doing, they have given widespread legitimacy to an array of mind/body techniques that are helping change the face of medicine.

The Mind/Body Connection to Fertility

All medical problems are potentially stressful. But few tap into women's anxieties as deeply as infertility.

A growing body of science is finding links between emo-tional health and the ability to conceive. Given the compli-cated nature of reproduction, this is hardly surprising. Yet the idea that women can "think" or "feel" their way to improved fertility is just starting to gain wider acceptance.

Mind/body medicine seeks to correct emotional imbalances that may be contributing to conception problems. This can be done in numerous ways, from breathing exercises to hypnosis to guided imagery. These techniques are often used in conjunction with other therapies, both conventional and alternative. Indeed, although few doctors treat infertility solely through stress management, more and more practitioners understand that reducing stress, depression, and other emotional problems can enhance fertility.

Much of the emphasis of mind/body medicine in relation to fertility is on hormonal balance. "Being able to enter a state of deep relaxation helps physiologically in terms of the mechanics of hormone release and ovulatory cycles," says Joel M. Evans, M.D., who as founder and director of the Center for Women's Health in Darien, Connecticut, uses a variety of mind/body techniques to treat infertility. "One of the things you learn early on in obstetrics and gynecology is that stress is one of the most common reasons for abnormal periods. One reason for that is interruption of the very delicate hormonal balance between the hypothalamus, the pituitary, and the ovaries. By spending more and more time in a relaxed state, we can restore that delicate balance."

While science has established a clear link between stress and reproductive hormonal imbalance, a lot remains unknown about how the mind/body approach works. "We have to understand that we won't understand every reason why these techniques are effective," states Dr. Evans. One reason, he says, is that mind/body medicine helps people to resolve conflicts in their lives, which in turn makes it easier to conceive. These techniques may also provide women with insight into conflicts that exist on a subconscious level. "When people are in a state of deep relaxation, they may come up with an awareness of conflict in an area they thought was calm, such as dissatisfaction with career or lack of creativity or something they thought was not important and all of a sudden they realize it's important," says Dr. Evans.

Acquiring methods for controlling your anxieties provides not only a sense of empowerment but often a real improvement in the quality of your life. In some cases, it may help save relationships jeopardized by the pressures of infertility. In others, it may foster a deepened commitment or intimacy that enhances the process of seeking conception.

Whether it directly increases your chances of getting pregnant, gives you the tools to better manage your stress, or both, mind/body medicine is a key part of a natural fertility program.

LESS STRESS, MORE CONTROL

Most of us have firsthand knowledge of how the mind can affect the body—in good and bad ways. Many people, for instance, succumb to flus or colds during bouts of depression. And almost everyone has seen what a little relaxation can do for a tension headache.

Mind/body medicine recognizes that such experiences are not coincidental. Instead, it views the interaction of the physical and mental/emotional realms as the foundation upon which our total health rests.

Certain principles are central to the mind/body approach. The first one is that psychological and emotional stress affects our physical well-being. Thus, much of mind/body medicine is devoted to reducing stress as a way of preventing or treating illness.

While professional assistance can be helpful in learning stress-reduction techniques, mind/body medicine embraces the idea that we can help to heal ourselves. This is a departure from much of Western medicine, which has tended to regard patients the way parents see children—as powerless agents dependent upon them for survival. The mind/body approach understands the critical role played by doctors, but also places equal responsibility on individuals to maintain or restore health by tending to emotional as well as physical needs.

Mind/Body Fertility Pioneers: Alice Domar and Niravi Payne

Alice Domar, Ph.D., of Boston, Massachusetts, has been dubbed the fertility goddess in the national press. And no wonder: nearly half the women who complete her mind/body program get pregnant within 6 months. The numbers are even higher—55%—for those who participated in Dr. Domar's 5-year National Institute of Mental Health study.

The truly amazing thing about these figures, however, is that pregnancy is not the goal of Dr. Domar's mind/body program. Her objective is to help women deal with the stress and depression that often accompany infertility. It just so happens that, as these women recover their emotional health, they keep getting pregnant.

Meanwhile, in New York, Niravi B. Payne, M.S., has spent more than a decade developing a highly successful natural fertility program based on mind/body practices. Hailed by acclaimed author Dr. Christiane Northrup as the creator of "a whole new language and approach to fertility," Payne has taught her techniques to hundreds of women.

In 1987, Dr. Domar began working with women who had been trying unsuccessfully for 2 years or more to get pregnant with the aid of high-tech procedures. Sponsored by the Harvard University–affiliated Beth Israel Deaconess Medical Center in Boston, the program was designed to help participants deal with the emotional aspects of infertility through stress reduction. It didn't take long, however, for Dr. Domar to observe that upon learning techniques to manage depression and anxiety, many of the women were conceiving.

Nearly a decade later, Dr. Domar, again with Harvard's support, started the Mind/Body Center for Women's Health, which offers programs for infertility along with menopause, chronic fatigue syndrome, and other conditions. She has documented her groundbreaking work on the relationship between emotional and physical health in *Healing Mind, Healthy Woman,* which explains how mind/body medicine can help women with everything from infertility to eating disorders to breast cancer.

Dr. Domar's work has had a noticeable ripple effect. "We're seeing tremendously increased interest by physicians and nurses," she says. "We have affiliates around the United States, and more and more are picking up infertility."

Payne, a psychotherapist and biofeedback specialist, became interested in infertility in the early 1980s, when a client's struggle to conceive touched a personal chord. As Payne explains in her book *The Whole Person Fertility Program*SM, she had had difficulty conceiving herself some 40 years earlier. Using her counseling skills and knowledge of mind/body medicine, she was able to help the woman get pregnant. This experience and others like it prompted her to create a center devoted to natural fertility in Brooklyn Heights, New York.

Payne has developed a 10-step program that combines many common mind/body practices, such as relaxation and visualization, with other exercises that focus on emotional healing. For example, she has clients look at family photos as a way of connecting with their emotional history. In another exercise, clients strengthen or repair relationships with their mothers by expressing to themselves feelings about pregnancy, motherhood, and other issues. Such techniques are part of a process she calls "conscious conception."

"The process of conscious conception entails a willingness to understand the origin of the negative messages that your mind is communicating to your body," writes Payne in her book. "Your body communicates to you through physical symptoms, particularly as reproductive difficulties. Conscious conception means that you deliberately use your mind to translate the physical symptoms, particularly blocks to conception, by identifying and releasing deeply held unexpressed emotions."

Mind/Body Techniques to Reduce Stress: Two Approaches

Interest in the connection between mind/body techniques and infertility has continued to grow, with programs being started every day. Here are two examples of how the mind/body approach is being used with women seeking to get pregnant.

Alice Domar and the Beth Israel Mind/Body Medical Clinic

Since beginning her pioneering mind/body work in 1987, Dr. Domar has seen hundreds of women go through her program. The typical patient is in her mid- to late 30s, basically healthy, and has been trying to get pregnant for about 3 years, often through high-tech procedures. She works as a professional and tends to be a perfectionist.

"Infertility is making her crazy," says Dr. Domar. "She hates everyone who is pregnant, she and her husband are fighting, she doesn't understand why he doesn't feel the same, and will do anything to get pregnant, yet is afraid of the side effects of treatment. She comes to the program when she's hit bottom. She's miserable, with a lot of physical symptoms such as headaches, insomnia, abdominal pain. She's having a hard time at work and is really wondering what to do if she can't get pregnant. She's angry and depressed and sad."

Once they enter the program, the changes these women undergo are dramatic, says Dr. Domar. "Within a couple of weeks they start to laugh, and week by week their old self reemerges. By the tenth week you hear them say, 'This is who I am.' They're really able to control their lives again. I've been doing this for twelve years, and it still absolutely stuns me looking at the difference in their faces at the first session and the last."

Dr. Domar's program consists of 2 individual sessions and 10 group sessions. At the first visit, women fill out a lengthy questionnaire covering a wide range of issues, including their infertility history, medical background, psychological history, social support, and health habits. After the final group session, participants have a discharge assessment.

Each woman is assigned a partner. While this buddy system is usually based on geography, sometimes the participants with a similar background—recurrent miscarriage, for example— are paired.

The typical group session begins with a half-hour of optional sharing. Then the women break into small discussion groups while Dr. Domar reads the diaries they bring in. This is followed by a brief lecture on a chosen theme. The next step is small-group exercises, after which comes a large-group discussion, with a 2-minute relaxation exercise to conclude the session. Graduates of previous programs act as co-leaders, providing an experiential perspective and serving as role models for others.

There are six components to Dr. Domar's program.

RELAXATION RESPONSE

This part of the program involves teaching women different relaxation techniques. Dr. Domar provides participants with audiotapes and advises them to listen 20 minutes a day. She also shows them how to do mini-relaxation exercises, such as focused breathing, that they can use during infertility treatment.

APPROPRIATE NUTRITION

Since diet is such an important issue in conception, Dr. Domar offers women a primer on nutrition, discussing how such factors as caffeine, weight, folic acid and calcium, and vitamins can affect fertility. She also addresses the question of exercise, and although suggesting that patients stop vigorous exercising for 3 months, her center does teach yoga.

COGNITIVE RESTRUCTURING

This method controls negative thoughts. Typical examples, says Dr. Domar, include "I'll never have a baby," "My husband will leave me if I don't get pregnant," "God's punishing me," "I'll be a terrible mother," and "I shouldn't have had an abortion." By asking patients questions that challenge these ideas, she helps them to restructure their thinking. For instance, if a woman has had a miscarriage, often she'll say that God is punishing her. "I say, 'You think God kills babies?' And they say, 'Of course not.' So they end up saying they don't know why they're miscarrying."

EMOTIONAL EXPRESSION

Learning how to handle negative emotions is a key part of Dr. Domar's approach. She focuses particularly on anger. "Most women are taught they are not allowed to get angry when they're kids," she explains. "Women are made angry by infertility and don't know what to do with that. Anger is a very healthy emotion. We teach them ways to be angry that don't push people away."

SOCIAL SUPPORT

Women dealing with infertility often experience devastating isolation. "Most have siblings, friends, and co-workers who get pregnant, and they feel very isolated from them," says Dr. Domar. "We talk about how they can get more support in their lives and how to cope with people in the fertile world."

SELF-NURTURING

The program also emphasizes the importance of taking care of yourself—something that frequently goes by the wayside for women struggling to get pregnant. "Women stop buying themselves clothes, stop having fun because they are so miserable," says Dr. Domar.

Dr. Domar identifies three major shifts that occur in the women who go through her program. First, by being with other women going through the same experience, they gain a sense of reassurance. Second, by learning the relaxation techniques, they calm down. Third, through the cognitive restructuring, they start to challenge the devastating self-critical thinking that frequently accompanies infertility.

The other change that takes place for many of the women is that they get pregnant. Conception rates for graduates of the program seem tied to the level of emotional duress they're under when they begin. "The more distressed the woman is when she comes into the program, the more likely she is to get pregnant. If distress is contributing to infertility, then if it goes away, it makes sense that she's more likely to get pregnant." She notes that women who are not depressed when they start the program have a 25% rate of pregnancy within 6 months of graduation, while the figure for those who come in very depressed is a stunning 60%.

Joel Evans and the Center for Women's Health

As director of the Center for Women's Health in Darien, Connecticut, Dr. Joel Evans has treated a lot of women for infertility. Over the years, he has witnessed the emotional strain suffered by many of these patients.

"I saw that infertility issues created a lot of stress in patients and their marriages, and that the ones that were able to handle that stress were to my observation getting pregnant faster," says Dr. Evans. "I also observed that very stressful lives—either from personal, emotional, family, marital, or financial issues— also contributed to difficulties conceiving. From that observation I wanted to educate myself about stress reduction."

Dr. Evans took a course in mind/body medicine and started applying the techniques to his own life. Then he began to incorporate this approach into his practice, creating a mind/body skills group. As in Dr. Domar's program, the subsequent pregnancy rates have been eye-opening.

"Dr. Domar's work has confirmed what I've seen in my practice," he says. "I have a two-thirds success rate for pregnancy in the mind/body skills group. Most of the women are end line, where the chances of the medical treatment working is described by physicians as minimal. They've usually tried one or two cycles of fertility treatments, sometimes more, without success. Some have success without medical techniques. Others use techniques that haven't worked in the past."

Dr. Evans uses a number of techniques, including the following:

DRAWINGS

Women are asked to draw pictures depicting their greatest problems. "Some of them will draw an empty family. Others might draw a relationship with an abusive or absent parent." One woman drew a picture of her mother, and was struck by the thought that her mother had died during childbirth. "Of course, she knew this already, but with the drawing she realized that she had some fear about herself dying during childbirth," explains Dr. Evans. "By seeing this on paper, she had an awareness that this was creating ambivalence in her desire to conceive." The woman was then able to discuss the issue, both in a group setting and in one-on-one counseling. She later went on to conceive.

How can feelings such as fear or ambivalence prevent conception? "Physiologically, I think what that does is during intercourse, when they're trying to conceive, she secretes some stress hormones, and those hormones then interfere with the mechanism that allows the sperm to penetrate. The fallopian tubes have little fine hairs called cilia, and they propel both the sperm and fertilized egg. I believe when she secretes these stress hormones, they then act on the cilia and fallopian tubes and decrease their effectiveness." Dr. Evans adds that stress hormones might also prevent ovulation from occurring.

IMAGERY

This technique begins with relaxation exercises. "Once you enter a deeply relaxed state, you are open to receiving feedback about different parts of the body," says Dr. Evans. "I'll say, 'Let's focus on your breathing—how does it feel? Then we spend a lot of time on the reproductive organs, and sometimes get a sense from that if there's a problem." He recalls the case of a woman who, after having a body scan, said she felt a lot of heat coming from one ovary. Dr. Evans recommended that the woman see her regular doctor to check. "Sure enough, she ended up having a cyst on her ovary."

RELAXATION

The goal here is to get the body to enter a parasympathetic state. The simplest way to do this is with belly breathing, says Dr. Evans, which involves closing your eyes while sitting in a comfortable position or lying down, then taking slow, deep breaths. You must use your diaphragm to breathe. To check, put your hand on your belly; your hand should go up and down. This type of breathing stimulates the vagus nerve, or parasympathetic nerve, which runs through the diaphragm. "While you're doing that, you can think of a word or phrase that is relaxing: love, peace, everything is okay, whatever. For fertility we might say, 'I am open to conceive.'" Relaxation not only lowers the heart rate and blood pressure and enhances immune cell function, it also helps restore the delicate hormonal balance between the hypothalamus and the pituitary. "That balance is easily thrown off by stress," explains Dr. Evans.

AUTOGENICS

Autogenics involves the silent, mouthed repetition of certain phrases that can affect the physiology of specific body parts. For example, "My hands are heavy and warm." There are 10 classic autogenic phrases. "If you repeat it six or seven times in a deeply relaxed state, they have documented increased blood flow to the body part you're describing," says Dr. Evans. "We use that to increase blood flow to the reproductive organs." He uses phrases specific to conception: "The circulation to my pelvis is strong and healthy," "My ovaries are fertile," "My uterus is receptive to a pregnancy." By increasing blood flow, the health of these organs is enhanced.

VISUALIZATION

This exercise entails creating a whole script about the conception process, then reciting it. Although each narrative is individualized, it might begin something like this, says Dr. Evans: "I'm very much in love with my husband and with the idea of being a mother. I'm devoted to family and grounded in the earth and in community. I want to form my own little community." Then the women are directed to visualize the act of creating new life. "Imagine sperm traveling through the vagina, the cervix, the uterus, the fallopian tubes, the egg releasing, the two of them meeting, the light surrounding that, the power, the spark of life from the universe bathing this newly formed embryo in light and love. Imagine the embryo implanting in the uterus and growing, connecting with the mother's blood supply in a healthy way, growing to be a baby, and then being delivered."

The first goal of visualization is to put the women into a relaxed state. But it also puts them into a state of mind where they can more easily imagine being pregnant and being a parent. "There's no scientific way to evaluate or prove this," says Dr. Evans. "It's based on the concept of intent being important. I believe very much in the value of intent being important in achieving an outcome."

If a woman is experiencing infertility due to a specific condition, Dr. Evans will encourage her to address the problem directly with her thoughts. Here are a few examples.

ENDOMETRIOSIS
"I would like all of the old cells to come out from below and for none of the old cells to go backward into my pelvis."

HORMONAL IMBALANCE
"I would like my hypothalamus and pituitary to relax in a way that is healthy."

POLYCYSTIC OVARIES
"I would like the cyst to go away and the ovaries to produce hormones in a healthy way."

BIOFEEDBACK
Years before mind/body medicine became an established field, this method of controlling various physical functions was being explored. Biofeedback is the practice of sending low-range electronic stimulation through the body to encourage the body's own systems to work more efficiently. Dr. Evans uses biofeedback early on in his workshops to demonstrate to patients that they can regulate their physiology. He hooks them up to monitors that measure temperature in the fingers, showing them how the reading goes up with positive emotions and down with negative ones. "By proving it to people right then and there in the group, they believe there is worth to this." Later, they can use the monitors to gauge the effectiveness of exercises focused on the reproductive organs.

Other Mind/Body Approaches to Infertility

When it comes to relieving the stress that goes along with trying to have a baby, finding someone who understands can be invaluable. Laura Kaufman, M.F.C.T., of Sherman Oaks, California, is a therapist who specializes in infertility counseling. It's a subject she knows something about, having had two miscarriages and numerous rounds of high-tech treatment before finally delivering a healthy child. Prior to the conception that led to the healthy birth, Kaufman started using visualization and self-hypnosis. "I can't tell you why I got pregnant, but I know that after I did those exercise I felt better, it was easier to cope," she says.

Now Kaufman teaches those techniques to her clients. Before she does that, however, she helps them understand the emotional stress that in many cases is taking over their lives. "I try to find out what's going on and demystify some of the process," explains Kaufman.

One of the keys, she says, is convincing the women that it's okay to feel what they feel—despite what others or their own critical inner voices may say. For instance, many women struggling with infertility would prefer not to go to baby showers. "I say, 'You're not being selfish, you're taking care of yourself.' We're assaulted by all the visual stuff about babies and families. When you say, 'I don't have to do this,' it takes away some of the stress."

Kaufman also counsels the women about the importance of paying attention to their needs. "What happens with infertility is they deprive themselves, which causes stress too. You have to have a life, do things to nurture yourself." She notes that women trying to get pregnant often avoid changes in their lives—from new jobs to new clothes—putting everything on hold until later.

Kaufman supplies her clients with creative visualization tapes that they can use at home. The tapes begin with relaxation exercises, then offer affirming images of a fertilized egg and the various stages of pregnancy. "I never guarantee it will get you pregnant, but I guarantee you'll feel better."

She also uses hypnosis along with visualization. The idea,

says Kaufman, is to penetrate the unconscious with positive thoughts. "When you've [been trying to get pregnant] for years, there's this whole thing of 'Why am I doing this? It's not going to work.' When you get in there and give them a vision of something different, it helps them to relax, to think there's a different possibility."

Kaufman teaches interested clients how to use self-hypnosis. The process is relatively simple: you lay down in a comfortable position, hands on your thighs. Then you repeat certain words for different areas of the body. "I try to give my upper body the word 'confident,' my lower body the word 'floating,' then up around my head and eyes I give myself the words 'deep sleep.'" As your body relaxes, you visualize positive images in your mind. "You have to practice it. The more you do it, the more comfortable you get and the deeper state of relaxation you can go to. It gives you a sense of having control when you have no control. You can't make yourself get pregnant, but you can help yourself get calm."

Susan M. Lark, M.D., a prominent physician in the field of women's health, has observed a strong connection between stress and two leading causes of infertility: endometriosis and fibroid tumors. According to Dr. Lark, stress-related hormonal imbalances may aggravate endometriosis, and fibroid tumors grow during periods of stress.

Dr. Lark has developed a stress-reduction program specifically for women suffering from these conditions. Her regimen—outlined in her book *The Fibroid Tumors and Endometriosis Self-Help Book*—includes such relaxation exercises as focusing, meditation, progressive muscle relaxation, affirmations, and visualization. She also uses hydrotherapy, sound therapy, and biofeedback.

Dr. Lark's focusing exercises are designed to shift a woman's attention away from her pelvic area, with the goal of lowering discomfort and anxiety. Meditation also offers a way to reduce tension, and the physical distress that often goes with it, by clearing the mind. Muscle relaxation combats stress by targeting the area of tension and then retraining the body to let go of that tension. Affirmations and visualization use positive thinking to restore hormonal balance, while both hydrotherapy and sound therapy have a general relaxing effect.

"My patients have been very enthusiastic about the results they attain through stress-reduction exercise," writes Dr. Lark in her book. "They often tell me that they feel much calmer and happier. They also find their physical health improves. A calm mind seems to have beneficial effects on the body's physiology and chemistry, restoring the body to a normal condition."

Getting Started with Mind/Body Medicine

There are many ways to reduce stress and anxiety. Some are simple, whereas others require a bit more time and concentration. Many of these techniques can be learned and practiced on your own. However, you may find it more beneficial to work with a practitioner or join a program where you can share your experience with other women.

Here are examples of a relaxation exercise and a visualization you can do right away. Before starting, find a quiet place where you won't be interrupted. Wear loose-fitting clothes, and choose a position where you are comfortable but won't fall asleep.

RELAXATION

The following exercise, which takes about 20 minutes, is recommended by Dr. Domar in her book *Healing Mind, Healthy Woman*. It is designed to facilitate a richer intake of air and oxygen, which triggers the relaxation response.

Begin with a normal breath. Then take a deep, slow breath,

letting the air go through your nose and move into your lower stomach. Allow your stomach to expand as you breathe. Exhale through your mouth.

Now alternate one normal breath with one deep, abdominal breath. Notice the difference between the normal and the deep breaths as you inhale and exhale. Continue with deep breathing only, letting your stomach expand as it will. When you exhale, sigh. As you breathe, imagine that the air you're inhaling brings peace and calm and that the air you're exhaling is carrying away tension.

VISUALIZATION

This exercise is intended to create a sense of calm and well-being. Begin with a few minutes of slow, deep breathing. Close your eyes and imagine you are in a quiet, beautiful place—the beach, a forest, a river. In your mind, look around and notice the scenery. Focus on the details of color and shape and texture. Breathe in the smells and listen to the sounds of nature. Let your body feel the ripple of the wind, the warmth of the sun, the softness of the grass. If you want, imagine exploring the environment, lingering to stare at a flower or examine a pebble.

In our Resources section, you'll find various information that will help you learn more about putting mind/body principles to work. Like thousands of other women, you'll discover that restoring emotional health through stress reduction can help pave the way for pregnancy.

CHAPTER TEN

Keeping Your Sex Drive Active

In almost every relationship, lovemaking has its highs and lows. Sure, there's that honeymoon period where it seems like sexual thirst for your partner will never be quenched. But sooner or later, the erotic fires usually cool down a bit.

While many of us think back fondly on the passion that marked the first weeks or months of long-term relationships, in truth the tempering of sexual desire is a natural development. As the bond with your partner deepens, lovemaking takes its place alongside other aspects of the life you share together. And although you may not spend as much time in the bedroom, in good relationships the quality of that time continues to improve, bringing you closer to one another.

Of course, keeping your sex life active and interesting can be a challenge. This is true even under the best circumstances. And in the face of everyday inconveniences, or more serious issues such as career uncertainty, family turmoil, and health problems, lovemaking is often the first thing to suffer.

Perhaps the most common culprit when it comes to sexual problems is stress. It is one of the ironies of our age that even as technology provides us with more and more tools to make our lives more comfortable, tension and anxiety seem to be more rampant than ever.

One of the greatest sources of stress that any woman can encounter is infertility. So it's no surprise that the sex lives of couples trying to have a baby frequently succumb to the enormous pressures that go along with it.

In this chapter, we'll look at some of the issues that can interfere with healthy, fulfilling lovemaking. We'll discuss how sexual problems can actually contribute to infertility and why it's so important to work on these difficulties. We'll also offer a range of ideas on how to maintain or revive your sex life, as well as instructions on how to maximize the chances of conception after intercourse.

Making Love Versus Making Babies

While sexual problems may precede infertility, in most cases the stress of trying to get pregnant leads to difficulties in the bedroom. Performance anxiety, loss of spontaneity, overwhelming expectations—all take their toll on the lovemaking process.

"Sex for procreation is different than sex for recreation in terms of the sexual script," says Sandra Leiblum, Ph.D., a renowned specialist in the area of sexuality and infertility who teaches at the Robert Wood Johnson Medical School in Piscataway, New Jersey. "Seduction, taking time for foreplay, trying to make it mutually gratifying for both partners become less significant than having a successful ejaculation at ovulation. It's two very different ways of approaching intimacy."

Maintaining sexual intimacy and pleasure while trying to conceive requires a real commitment. Both partners must be sensitive to the needs of the other and must strive to prevent sex from being solely about conceiving a child. For women, that means being careful not to treat their mates like a sperm bank. "People have got to keep clear in their mind that they are there with their partner, their partner is not just a sperm deliverer, which is what guys sometimes end up feeling like," says Los Angeles, California–based author and sex educator L. Lou Paget, who teaches workshops that offer practical ideas on how to keep sex exciting.

Paget observes that while trying to get pregnant can put a strain on lovemaking, in many cases it simply exposes problems that have been swept under the sheets. "Lack of spontaneity and creativity just about invariably happen in every long-term relationship. Attributing it to just wanting to have a child is shining a light in the wrong direction of the room. It may contribute to it, but it's not the only factor." She advises couples to be honest with each other about sexual issues that may arise when they are trying to conceive.

Often the experience of a professional counselor can be invaluable in helping people work through sexual issues. Bryce Britton, M.F., of Santa Monica, California, is a sex therapist who has worked with many couples experiencing fertility problems. She says one of the first things she does is establish some consensus on what her clients want from their sex lives. "The one goal that I set is that both of them leave the lovemaking situation feeling good about themselves and their partner."

After meeting separately with each partner and taking a sexual history, Britton begins the process of reestablishing a strong foundation for sexual intimacy. The first step is simple breathing techniques. "The breath is the bridge that connects the body to the mind, and that change doesn't happen just by talking," explains Britton. The exercises work on the autonomic nervous system, which controls human sexual response, and are designed to help the couples relax as well as bring them back into their bodies.

Next, Britton takes her clients through a series of face and hand caresses, with one partner receiving and the other giving. The idea is to break down the sexual arousal process and reintroduce them to the act of giving pleasure to each other. "Even though there's this urgency to have intercourse, I ask them to practice these exercises when they're not in ovulation mode to build a firmer foundation so they can have more intimate bonding when it comes to that get-it-on time," states Britton.

Britton also works with the couples on transitioning from foreplay to intercourse without losing the sexual excitement or the intimacy. At the end of these sessions, both partners offer their feedback on what they liked and what they didn't like. "A lot of people have never done this. We're creating a new way for them to be sexual partners together."

Addressing underlying emotional issues is another essential part of dealing with sexual problems. "I urge communication," says Sharon Siegel, Ph.D, of West Hollywood, California, who has worked with infertile couples for the past 25 years. She has found that resolving difficulties unrelated to sex is often the key to better lovemaking. "Hold the relationship sacred and work towards an everybody-wins solution," advises Dr. Siegel.

Every couple must decide for themselves whether to seek counseling, and it's best not to wait until the relationship has sustained serious damage. If a deep rift develops between you and your partner, not only will your sex life suffer but the resulting stress will make it that much harder to get pregnant.

Sexual Dysfunction and Fertility

Sex, as everyone knows, can lead to pregnancy. But lack of knowledge about sex can lead to infertility. The same is true of sexual dysfunction.

How common is the link between sexual problems and infertility? "I think it's more frequent than we are often aware of," says Linda Hammer Burns, Ph.D., who teaches at the University of Minnesota Medical School in Minneapolis and is a leading authority in the field of infertility counseling.

According to Dr. Hammer Burns, sexual dysfunction may be traced to physical, emotional, or psychological issues. In many cases, people are aware of the situation, but often they aren't. Problems can range from infrequent intercourse to excessive masturbation by the male to ambivalence by either partner.

"Sometimes couples are undereducated about what it takes for reproduction," states Dr. Hammer Burns. "The biggest factor is one partner is aware and the other is not."

When counseling couples who are experiencing infertility, Dr. Hammer Burns takes an extensive history to determine if sexual dysfunction may be contributing to the woman's inability to get pregnant. She inquires about sexual or physical abuse, trauma associated with past pregnancies, and sexually transmitted diseases (STDs). These issues can potentially have serious effects on a woman's fertility, either by making sexual intercourse emotionally difficult or, in the case of STDs, by interfering with healthy reproductive function.

How to Rev Up Your Sex Life

There are numerous factors that can put a damper on lovemaking. But there are just as many ways to get your sex drive back in high gear. Here are some suggestions that can help.

VARYING THE LOCATION

An often overlooked way to keep lovemaking fresh is to change the location. Rather than confining it to your bedroom, try to find alternatives such as the living room couch, the rug in front of the fireplace, or even the kitchen counter. Taking it out of the house altogether is a good way to relax as well as perk things up. Go on a vacation or visit a resort. Even arranging a night in a nearby hotel will help you to leave behind thoughts about bills, job pressures, and other day-to-day concerns. If you and your partner enjoy risk-taking, having sex in unusual places can be stimulating.

Some people like the freedom of making love outside in nature. Try a camping trip, or if your backyard is private enough, there's nothing wrong with experimenting there. Remember that intercourse does not have to be the goal. After a few minutes of kissing and touching in a dark movie theater, the prospect of getting home and into bed can be exciting. Just beginning the process in a different location can reenergize lovemaking for you and your partner.

Although physical location is important, Britton observes that the greatest obstacle to passionate sex is sometimes in our head. "The big challenge is to change the setting in your own mind. When you come together there can be a silent period where maybe you just hug and take some time for each person. It's the mental stuff that keeps us trapped in thinking that the person was the way they were that morning."

CHANGING THE ROUTINE

The very things that make having sex with the same partner for a long time such a pleasurable experience—comfort, familiarity, knowing their likes and dislikes—can also lead to stagnancy. When this happens, changing the routine can make a huge difference. Start with shifting the responsibility of lovemaking from one person to the other. For example, if the man is usually the one who indicates interest, the woman should try being aggressive. If the woman likes morning sex but her partner is a night person, he should make the effort to rouse himself early and get things going. Taking turns focusing on one partner at a time is also a good way to liven things up. Devise an entire session to pleasing just one of you—new things you want to try, your favorite positions, your orgasm.

Subtle changes in your routine can also have an impact. Try altering your rhythm or slowing things down. If both of you like sweet, tender lovemaking, experiment with passionate energy and hot, sweaty sex. These changes may feel strange at first, but they will broaden your sexual repertoire, and you may even discover that you prefer the new to the tried and true.

ATMOSPHERE

Setting the mood can make all the difference in lovemaking. Individual tastes vary, of course, but certain things seem to bring on that loving feeling in almost everybody. The right music can cast an erotic spell, whether it's Barry White, a Beethoven symphony, a bossa nova, or an African trance. Another favorite is candles. It's amazing what turning down the lights and letting the flames flicker can do. For many, incense heightens the effect. Another way to let fragrance set the stage for romance is aromatherapy (see "Aphrodisiacs"). Rub some onto your partner's body, or better yet, buy an aromatherapy bath preparation and crawl into the tub together. But don't forget to lock the door, feed the pets, and turn off the beeper and cell phone. There's nothing like last-second chores or interruptions to ruin a romantic rendezvous.

ATTIRE

It might seem ironic, but wearing sexy attire is one of the best ways to get your partner to tear your clothes off. Lingerie is a reliable turn-on for both sexes, but don't wait until you go to bed to let attire work its magic. Treat yourself to an occasional shopping spree that focuses on clothes that make you feel sexy. It's fun to surprise your partner with a new outfit, or you can also heat things up by going together and showing off the possibilities. When choosing your wardrobe, remember that variety is the spice of life.

APHRODISIACS

For thousands of years, human beings have been adding zest to lovemaking with natural stimulants. In her excellent book *Love Potions: A Guide to Aphrodisiacs and Sexual Pleasures*, Cynthia Watson, M.D., surveys a wide range of foods, herbs, and oils associated with pleasures of the flesh. They include the following:

Bananas   Loaded with potassium, which enhances nerve and muscle function, the phallically provocative banana is regarded as a sexual stimulant by numerous cultures.

Asparagus   This nutrient-rich vegetable is considered a kidney tonic by the Chinese, in whose system of medicine the kidneys regulate sexual desire.

Oysters   High in zinc and other nutrients, oysters have long been coveted for their aphrodisiacal powers.

Honey   This most sensual of natural sweeteners gains its erotic charge not only from the energy it packs but also from its color, taste, and texture.

Chocolate   Speaking of sweet sensations, chocolate for many is the ultimate aphrodisiac. And no wonder, with its combination of caffeine, sugar, and the natural stimulant phenylalanine.

(*Caution:* Some herbs should not be used during pregnancy or if certain health conditions are present. Consult your practitioner to make sure an herbal aphrodisiac is safe.)

Ginseng   Now popular in the West, ginseng has been used since ancient times by Asian cultures to boost sexual desire and performance. It does this not by impacting the reproductive system itself but by improving overall endurance.

Damiana   A sexual tonic for both men and women, damiana stimulates the nerves and reproductive organs and is known to produce erotic dreams.

Chasteberry In small amounts (3 to 6 grams daily), this herb can boost sexual desire.

Wild Yam Widely used to stabilize hormone levels, wild yam increases progesterone and testosterone.

Licorice Employed by various cultures to stimulate the sex drive, licorice contains chemicals that resemble those released by the adrenal glands.

(*Note:* See Chapter 7 for instructions on how to use aromatherapy remedies.)

Rose The mother of all scents, rose is revered, particularly by women, as one of the most potent aphrodisiacs in the natural kingdom.

Jasmine Another potent stimulant, jasmine is reputed to relieve impotence and frigidity.

Ylang-ylang The rich perfume of this flower is known to be intoxicating, relaxing the nerves.

Sandalwood A low-key aphrodisiac, sandalwood is considered a sexual tonic for both men and women.

Cardamom In seed form, it neutralizes the smell of garlic. Applied as an oil, cardamom ignites the fires of passion.

FLIRTING

Focusing on new ways or places to have intercourse isn't the only way to add spice to your sex life. Much of what people think of as intercourse really begins outside of the bedroom with the building of sexual tension. Erotic desire is created with looks, touches, and wordplay that often take place quite removed from any sexual activity. Flirting is a powerful psychological tool that both men and women can use to create anticipation. You can trigger what Britton calls "erotic simmering" by calling your partner during the day and letting him or her know you'll be in the mood that night.

Lovemaking can be enhanced by sensual but nonsexual activities including massages, cuddling, and holding hands. Touching your partner can be arousing even if you don't have intercourse until hours later. Try lightly trailing your fingertips along your partner's arms, running your fingers through your partner's hair, or blowing on his or her neck.

FOREPLAY

The initial stages of lovemaking sometimes go by the wayside when couples have been together a while, especially when one or both partners are under a lot of stress. Foreplay offers a great opportunity for playful intimacy that gets the libido rolling. Britton counsels couples to spend more time kissing and petting with their clothes on. "Try to re-create how it was when you were dating," she advises. "People tend to get stuck in their habits." Women in particular like light strokes and touching before things get hot and heavy.

If foreplay seems too predictable, mix it up. "It's important to have variety," says Britton. "I suggest experimenting with other things—mutual masturbation, oral sex—and be creative when you are pleasuring; use all different parts of your body." Women can pay more attention to often ignored erogenous zones such as a man's nipples and scrotum. Men can explore different ways to stimulate their partner's clitoris, including full lip contact or sucking rather than just licking.

NEW POSITIONS

Something as simple as experimenting with new positions can revitalize lovemaking between you and your partner. Sometimes all it takes is a small change—legs drawn together instead of spread apart, or tilting the body forward—to make a world of difference. The *Kama Sutra*, a guide to love and sex written in ancient India, is a good place to get inspiration, but you can come up with a lot of original ideas just by being creative and willing to laugh.

Most couples don't realize that even the standard missionary position—woman on her back, man on top—has numerous variations. If, for example, the woman usually bends her knees, with her feet on the mattress and her partner between her legs, she can try straightening her legs and squeezing them together. This increases the direct pressure on his penis and adds friction for her. She can bend her legs at the hips, drawing her knees up close to her chest, allowing for deeper penetration, or if she's really flexible, she can rest the backs of her legs against the man's shoulders.

The man can also breathe new life into the missionary position with a few adjustments. One variation is to lift his torso up by leaning on his hands, which alters the angle at which he enters his partner. If he's flexible, he can sit on his knees, tilting her buttocks up toward him and changing the angle even further. Another good idea is to try moving his whole body up a few inches from where it usually rests on her. This increases friction for him and helps his pubic bone rub directly on her clitoris, intensifying her pleasure.

Britton suggests a variation of the missionary position where the man's chest is more to one side rather than directly on top of his partner and his arms are underneath her. "Their pubic bones are more lined up so there's this rocking motion. There's not a lot of inside-outside thrusting, but grinding. Seventy-five to eighty percent of women can have a vaginal orgasm this way."

There are also many ways to play around with the rear-entry position, commonly known as "doggy style." Classically, the woman is on her hands and knees, while the man kneels behind her. You and your partner can take turns spreading or squeezing your legs together. Try lying flat, with the woman on her stomach, or rearing back with both partners kneeling.

Another opportunity for creativity is altering the standard woman-on-top position. Experiment with body angles and the directions your bodies move. The man can sit up so that he's face-to-face with his partner, or the woman can turn her body around to face away from him completely. Female-dominant positions offer wonderful freedom for touching, playing, and kissing each other.

Leaning against a bed or couch, with one person standing and the other sitting, works well. Lying on your sides, either facing one another or "spooning," is another option. Try this one standing in the shower: the woman bends at the hips, reaching as far down with her hands as she can, and the man stands behind her.

Not all of these positions will feel right to everybody, and, depending on how your bodies fit together, some may not even work. However, the sky is the limit here, so use your imagination and explore the possibilities.

PROPS

You and your partner may be able to generate all the excitement you need with your bodies alone. But it can be fun, and very stimulating, to experiment with sex toys and other objects. A good place to start is with vibrators, which many women find to be extremely pleasurable. Vibrators come in all shapes, sizes, and colors and can be used alone or with your partner. The selection of sex toys is virtually endless, and personal tastes vary greatly. Plan an outing together and find a few items that both of you like. "I have had several clients go to love boutiques that are a little softer than [most sex shops]," says Britton. "They have a friendly atmosphere that encourages the pleasure concept." Mail-order catalogs are also available if you prefer to do your erotic shopping in private.

Another option is to get creative at home. For some people, fruits, vegetables, and other foods offer a feast of sensory delight. Phallic-shaped produce such as carrots and zucchinis are an obvious option, but don't forget to explore the erotic possibilities of cherries, grapes, and berries. Others may go in for the pleasures of a feather massage, while a simple blindfold can heighten arousal for many. If you look around the house, you'll likely discover quite a few things that could be put to use in the bedroom. Choose a few in advance and try them out one by one. The element of surprise alone often is enough to get temperatures rising.

Many couples enjoy watching erotic videos together. In recent years, videos made by women have become available. "They're more for a woman's arousal pattern," notes Britton, "and not so focused on the genitals." Those looking to explore lovemaking with a spiritual dimension can rent tapes that offer instruction in the art of tantric sex.

By getting adventurous, couples sometimes discover that they have similar interests that have previously gone unexplored. Britton recounts the experience of a man and woman who had been married for 4 years. "He was very visual and liked to use pornography but had not shared that with her. It turned out that she had been reading a lot of erotica. They put that together and were able to use that in a very healthy way. He got what he wanted and she reached very high states of arousal."

FANTASIES

There's nothing like a good erotic fantasy to ignite the libido. Nearly everybody indulges in such flights of fancy, but most of us keep them to ourselves. Try sharing these sexual scenarios with your partner and vice versa. Better yet, you can create them together, improvising new adventures as a form of foreplay. If you need help getting started, there's plenty of good erotica to be found these days, much of it written by women (see Resources). "People can get in sync by reading erotica to each other," says Britton. "When a person does that and the other is listening, the actual brain waves become

208 GETTING PREGNANT THE NATURAL WAY

synchronized." Find a volume you like and read portions of it to your partner. You can even recite passages to each other during the initial stages of lovemaking, although eventually you'll want to put the book down and concentrate on the real thing.

Another option is audiotapes that use imagery to help couples break down barriers. "With a creative visualization where they imagine the body as a flowing rhythm, they can get into a trance state," explains Britton. "People become very relaxed and dreamlike, and are more receptive to giving or receiving touch." She recalls a couple who were having difficulty with physical intimacy and were able to reconnect with the help of a creative visualization tape. "They would get into a deep trance state, then they found a whole other level of erotic power."

THE LESS-IS-MORE APPROACH TO MALE SEXUAL VITALITY

In traditional Chinese medicine, it is believed that conserving male sexual energy is crucial to maintaining sexual health (see Chapter 3). The idea of forgoing ejaculation may initially strike most men as painful at best and unendurable at worst. But according to Roger Jahnke, O.M.D., L.Ac., of Santa Barbara, California, this chi gung practice can actually enhance a couple's lovemaking. "As people explore this process, they will discover another kind of orgasm experience that's multilevel," says Dr. Jahnke.

Ejaculation immediately saps most men of their sexual desire and often renders them less affectionate as well. Restraint, by contrast, allows a man to stay in a highly charged sexual state for longer, and, once his partner has climaxed, to engage in tender holding and caressing. For this reason, women value a man who is willing and able to hold back, says

Dr. Jahnke. "The guy not only performs the act to fulfill her desire for sexual outcome, but instead of ejaculating and losing his mind and falling asleep, he sustains a kind of affectionate presence following the consummation, and therefore the after-glow level is multiplied between 90% and 100%. Women like to have their men stay present and affectionate following sex, and if the guy ejaculates he's like a goner."

If this sounds like an act of male selflessness, it is not, assures Dr. Jahnke. Not only do men learn to take greater pleasure in satisfying their partners, but they experience a sense of fulfillment that comes from mastering the art of self-control. By refraining from ejaculation, they may also find that their libido increases, leading to more frequent and erotic lovemaking.

Chi gung sexual conservation takes practice. The most important skills to learn are breath control, relaxation, and mind-clearing. Dr Jahnke advises couples to be flexible and communicative; if holding back becomes physically uncom-fortable, a man should feel free to climax.

Ultimately, this technique is intended to help couples reach a higher level of both sexual and emotional intimacy. "If sex is just about ejaculation, the person you're with is getting the short end of everything," states Dr. Jahnke. "Is sex about ejac-ulating or about being in a relationship? Part of the retraining is to refocus oneself on making the relationship the primary focus of your sexual encounter."

Nutrition and Sex

Just as food affects fertility, it also affects sexual desire and per-formance. A whole-foods diet is a good place to start (see Chapter 6). According to Elson M. Haas, M.D., "Any diet . . . that maintains good circulation and normal weight and contains high-vitality fresh foods will lead to better sexual function."

Various nutrients have a direct effect on the organs and glands that control sexuality. The pituitary, for instance, is particularly sensitive to B vitamins, vitamin E, and zinc, while the adrenals depend on vitamin A, the B vitamins, vitamin C, vitamin E, and essential fatty acids. To keep the ovaries in prime condition, B vitamins, folic acid, vitamin E, and zinc are all important.

Although a healthy diet is always the first step when it comes to nutrition, supplementation may be needed not only for optimal fertility but also to maintain a healthy sexual drive. Dr. Watson recommends the following daily nutrient doses for women to attain optimum sexual function (nutrient doses for male sexual health are listed in Chapter 3):

B_1 50–200 milligrams

B_2: 50–200 milligrams

B_3: 50–500 milligrams

B_5: 50–1000 milligrams

B_6: 50–500 milligrams

B_{12}: 100–200 micrograms

Folic Acid: 800 micrograms

Choline: 500–3000 milligrams

Vitamin C: 1000–5000 milligrams

Bioflavonoids: 200–1000 milligrams

Vitamin A: 5000–10,000 international units

Beta-carotene: 15,000–25,000 international units

Vitamin E: 400–1000 international units

Calcium: 500–1500 milligrams

Magnesium: 500–1000 milligrams

Zinc: 30–50 milligrams

Selenium: 100–200 micrograms

Chromium: 200–500 micrograms

Iodine: 150 micrograms

Manganese: 10–15 milligrams

Iron: 20 milligrams

Phenylalanine: 500–1500 milligrams

Arginine: 100–1000 milligrams

Dr. Watson notes that arginine should be used with caution if you have herpes or other viral infections, and that iron supplementation is only necessary if you have a deficiency.

In his nutrient program for sexual vitality, Dr. Haas recommends the following daily supplements in addition to vitamins and minerals:

Flaxseed oil: 1–2 teaspoons

L-amino acids: 1000 milligrams

Inosine: 150–300 milligrams

Sex for Conception

One of the keys to keeping lovemaking fulfilling when you're trying to get pregnant is to focus on pleasure and intimacy. For most of your menstrual cycle, you should feel free to experiment with different styles and positions. During the days when you're fertile, however, you may want to use the positions that are more likely to lead to pregnancy. Niels H. Lauersen, M.D., recommends the following:

Missionary style

"Doggy Style"

Lying on your side

Dr. Lauersen advises against these positions for couples during the time of the month when they're trying to get pregnant:

Sitting

Standing

Female on top

Bending over

Fertility may be helped after intercourse by one of several things:

- Hold the lips of your vagina together for 5 to 10 minutes so that the sperm stay inside.
- Remain in a lying position for 15 to 20 minutes
- Lift your legs in the air or lean them against a wall.

Health writer Winifred Conkling offers some further suggestions to maximize the chances of conception. They include:

- Don't use oil-based or medicated vaginal lubricants.
- Have sex every other day.
- Use Robitussin (orally) for a few days before trying to conceive to increase fertile mucus (see Chapter 5 for more details).
- Don't have sex under water.
- Avoid douching.

Sex, Stimulants, and Medications— A Checklist

We're not always aware of how our habits and lifestyle can affect sexual vitality. Here are some substances—all of which were discussed in earlier chapters for their antifertility properties—that, according to Dr. Elson M. Haas, may compromise sexual desire and/or performance:

Alcohol

Nicotine

Coffee

Marijuana

Sugar

Tranquilizers

Anti-hypertensives

Birth control pills

If you or your partner is having sexual difficulties, consult with your practitioner to determine whether any of these substances may be contributing to the problem.

The Pleasure Principle

Does good sex increase the chance of getting pregnant? While fulfilling lovemaking is no guarantee, research suggests that greater sexual pleasure is a factor in fertility.

Dr. Lauersen points out that the hypothalamus, which plays a vital role in regulating hormonal function, functions better when we are feeling good than when we are upset or dissatisfied. In addition, he notes that passionate lovemaking ending in satisfying orgasm is one of the best ways to reduce stress, which as we've discussed can restore hormonal balance and thus contribute to optimal fertility.

Keeping your sex life active is its own reward. But mutually gratifying lovemaking is also an important part of a natural approach to fertility, providing a greater sense of physical and emotional well-being that will enrich your journey to motherhood.

Adoption and Other Alternatives

Infertility is a condition that lends itself to both tremendous hope and deep despair. Unless it's been determined that they absolutely cannot conceive, couples who want to have a child will frequently keep trying for years and years. Often their persistence is rewarded, but in many instances it is not.

The decision to consider other possibilities is a wrenching one. Yet at some point, you may face the prospect of deferring or giving up the dream of having your own child.

While the input of your health care practitioner is important, only you and your partner can determine when that time has come. Once you have, it can be helpful to know what your options are and how to start pursuing them.

While some infertile couples choose to forego parenting, many decide to adopt. Although the transition from trying to conceive to bringing an adopted child into your life is not easy, it offers millions of people a chance to fulfill their desire to have a family. Just as important, adoption can restore a sense of positive purpose for couples whose struggle to create a new life has resulted in pain and disappointment.

As with infertility, educating yourself about adoption is critical to a successful outcome. There are many issues to weigh, including cost, time, and legal protections. Couples also need to prepare themselves emotionally by examining their feelings about adoption, including hesitations they might have. Addressing these concerns early can be of great benefit to both you and your partner as well as your child.

GETTING STARTED

The first step is to learn as much as you can about the adoption process. There are many books on the subject, as well as Internet sites and organizations that provide information to the public (see Resources). By taking the time to familiarize yourself with the complexities of adoption, you will be in a better position to ask the right questions and avoid unanticipated problems.

AGENCY ADOPTION

One option for people wishing to adopt a child is to go through a state-licensed agency. In exchange for an agreed-upon fee, adoption agencies act as the liaison between the birth mother and the prospective parents.

There are two kinds of adoption agencies: private and public. In private agency adoption, an extensive home study is conducted before placement. This background check involves looking into every aspect of the adoptive family's life, from finances to health to criminal record.

In public agency adoption, a similar home study is done, but the cost is significantly less. The children tend to be older, and many come from the foster-care system.

One of the advantages of agency adoption, both private and public, is that the relinquishment agreement is more favorable to the adoptive parents. Also, public agencies charge their clients only if the adoption is finalized, while private agencies take part of the fee up front and the rest after the adoption is complete.

PRIVATE ADOPTION

You can also hire a lawyer to handle an adoption. Private adoption is often faster, in part because the home study is conducted after placement. As in agency adoption, the attorney receives a set fee for his or her services. However, the financial risk is greater, since the lawyer is paid whether or not the adoption goes through. And the cost is usually higher, as the adoptive family frequently must pay for the birth mother's health care, food, and housing expenses. Another consideration is the relinquishment agreement, which offers less protection than the one given to families by agencies.

INDEPENDENT ADOPTION

Some families arrange adoptions directly with the birth mother. Independent adoption has the advantage of being quicker and less bureaucratic. However, there are fewer legal safeguards. Not all states recognize independent adoptions, so it's essential to investigate the applicable laws before considering this approach.

INTERNATIONAL ADOPTION

Many couples choose to adopt children from other countries. This practice has become quite common in the last few decades, as people living in more affluent countries have become aware of the large number of parentless children abroad. International adoption is usually more complicated and time-consuming, as travel, language difficulties, foreign legal requirements, and other factors may be involved. It is also more expensive, since both the domestic and foreign adoption agencies charge a fee.

Open Versus Closed Adoption

Until fairly recently, most adoptions were closed. Under this system, information about a child's birth parents was sealed, and there was no contact between any of the parties involved. This practice, however, has come under increasing criticism, and an alternative—open adoption—has now become commonplace. While open adoption can take many different forms, it generally means that there is more contact between the parties involved and less effort to conceal the adoption from the child. The adoptive family often meets the birth mother during the pregnancy, and may even maintain contact after the baby is born. In other cases, families choose to give their adoptive child free access to information about his or her birth parents.

Cost

The cost of adopting a child varies widely. The average for private agency adoptions is around $10,000, whereas public agencies customarily charge significantly less. Adoptions handled by attorneys tend to be more expensive, although it depends on the circumstances.

Other Alternatives

There are several alternatives beyond adoption for infertile couples. Since these options are not the focus of this book, only a brief description follows. If you would like more information on either adoption or other alternatives to conventional pregnancy, see the Resources section.

Surrogacy

The use of surrogate mothers is relatively new and provides an option for couples when one or both partners are infertile. Surrogacy is a complex process, both logistically and emotionally, and should be weighed very carefully, ideally with the help of an experienced counselor.

DONOR EGG/SPERM

Some women choose to have the egg of another woman implanted in their uterus. In cases of male-factor infertility, fertilizing a woman's egg with sperm from another man offers a viable option. Again, it's important to consider all of the issues involved in these procedures before making a decision.

CHILD-FREE LIVING

Scientific advances have opened new paths to parenthood. But high-tech pregnancies are not for everyone. Many couples who are unable to have their own child decide to move on with their lives. Although abandoning the dream of parenthood may sound unfathomable, it is undoubtedly the right choice for some people. If one or both partners has been deeply traumatized by the experience of infertility, parenting a child who was adopted or born through egg/sperm donation or surrogacy may simply be too hard. In grappling with this question, the advice of a therapist is highly recommended. You and your partner may need to clarify some very sensitive issues, and a trained professional with experience in this area can provide much-needed insight, guidance, and support.

When and How to Approach Diagnostic Testing

The decision whether to undergo standard diagnostic testing for infertility depends on many factors. These include health, age, and how urgent your time frame is for having children.

Women under 35 who are in good health and have no significant menstrual problems generally can give themselves a year to get pregnant before considering testing. If you have one or more risk factors, such as a sexually transmitted disease, poor diet, and/or a high-stress lifestyle, you may want to consult with a practitioner prior to attempting conception. For women over 35, it's usually best to see a physician and assess possible obstacles to pregnancy. If there's a preexisting condition, doing some tests may keep you from wasting time and will help guide your treatment decisions.

A woman's symptoms and history will determine, in part, what tests are done. For example, if a woman has normal periods but an irregular ovulation pattern, it makes sense to check for anemia, thyroid problems, or polycystic ovaries. In cases of painful periods, endometriosis must be ruled out, while the possibility of narrowed fallopian tubes should be considered for those with sexually transmitted diseases (STDs) or endometriosis.

Test procedures vary widely. A blood test can gauge levels of such hormones as luteinizing hormone (LH), follicle-stimulating hormone (FSH), progesterone, estrogen, and prolactin, as well as thyroid function. Problems with cervical mucus can be detected with a postcoital test, which is administered in the doctor's office.

More sophisticated tests include the hysterosalpingogram, an x-ray procedure used to identify structural irregularities in the pelvis area. A falloposcopy utilizes an endoscope to view the uterus and fallopian tubes, while an ultrasound can reveal whether eggs are being produced and released. Other procedures, such as endometrial biopsy, culdoscopy, hysteroscopy, and laparoscopy, are more invasive.

One of the most basic tests is also one of the most useful: a semen sample. By examining sperm count, motility, shape, and other variables, many potential fertility issues can be ruled out. Men can also check their hormone levels with blood tests administered by their health professionals.

For both men and women, the standard diagnostic process includes a physical examination. Women are given a pelvic exam to inspect the cervix and look for potential uterine problems, while men are checked for abnormalities in the penis, testicles, or prostate.

Again, the question of pursuing diagnostic procedures is an individual one. Doing a whole battery of tests when there's little or no indication of serious fertility problems probably isn't necessary. However, in some cases such tests can be important in determining the cause of infertility.

Remember that the standard diagnostic workup can be used

in conjunction with alternative remedies. For example, if blood tests reveal a hormonal imbalance that's interfering with ovulation, dietary changes and herbal formulas may be able to correct the situation. This approach may prove to be the best for some people, combining the strengths of Western medicine and holistic therapies.

Sources

Introduction   The Path to Fertility

RESOLVE staff. *Resolving Infertility: Understanding the Options and Choosing the Solutions When You Want to Have a Baby.* New York: HarperCollins Publishers, 1999.

Chapter 1   What Is Infertility?

Northrup, Christiane. *Women's Bodies, Women's Wisdom: Creating Physical and Emotional Health and Healing.* New York: Bantam Books, 1998.

RESOLVE staff. *Resolving Infertility: Understanding the Options and Choosing the Solutions When You Want to Have a Baby.* New York: HarperCollins Publishers, 1999.

Chapter 2   The Menstrual Cycle—What Really Happens and What Can Go Wrong

Lauersen, Niels H., and Colette Bouchez. *Getting Pregnant: What Couples Need to Know Right Now.* New York: Fawcett Columbine, 1991.

Marrs, Richard, Lisa Friedman Bloch, and Kathy Kirtland Silverman. *Richard Marrs' Fertility Book: America's Leading Infertility Expert Tells You Everything You Need to Know About Getting Pregnant.* New York: Delacorte Press, 1997.

Northrup, Christiane. *Women's Bodies, Women's Wisdom: Creating Physical and Emotional Health and Healing.* New York: Bantam Books, 1998.

Chapter 3   Male Fertility

Conkling, Winifred. *Getting Pregnant Naturally: Healthy Choices to Boost Your Chances of Conceiving Without Fertility Drugs.* New York: Avon Books, 1999.

Lauersen, Niels H., and Colette Bouchez. *Getting Pregnant: What Couples Need to Know Right Now.* New York: Fawcett Columbine, 1991.

Marrs, Richard, Lisa Friedman Bloch, and Kathy Kirtland Silverman. *Richard Marrs' Fertility Book: America's Leading Infertility Expert Tells You Everything You Need to Know About Getting Pregnant.* New York: Delacorte Press, 1997.

Murray, Michael T., and Joseph Pizzorno. *Encyclopedia of Natural Medicine.* Rocklin, Calif.: Prima Publishing, 1998.

Watson, Cynthia Mervis. *Love Potions: A Guide to Aphrodisiacs and Sexual Pleasures.* New York: Tarcher/Putnam, 1993.

Wesson, Nicki. *Enhancing Fertility Naturally: Holistic Therapies for a Successful Pregnancy.* Rochester, Vt.: Healing Arts Press, 1997.

Chapter 5   How to Tell When You're Ovulating

Conkling, Winifred. *Getting Pregnant Naturally: Healthy Choices to Boost Your Chances of Conceiving Without Fertility Drugs.* New York: Avon Books, 1999.

Lauersen, Niels H., and Colette Bouchez. *Getting Pregnant: What Couples Need to Know Right Now.* New York: Fawcett Columbine, 1991.

Northrup, Christiane. *Women's Bodies, Women's Wisdom: Creating Physical and Emotional Health and Healing.* New York: Bantam Books, 1998.

Chapter 6   Eating and Supplementation for Natural Conception

Bolumar, F., J. Olsen, M. Rebagliato, L. Bisanti, and the European Study Group on Infertility and Subfecundity, Caffeine Intake and Delayed Conception. "A European Multicenter Study on Infertility and Subfecundity." *American Journal of Epidemiology*, v. 145 (4), February 15, 1997, pp. 324–334.

Bradstreet, Karen. *Overcoming Infertility Naturally: The Relationship Between Nutrition, Emotions and Reproduction.* Pleasant Grove, Utah: Woodland Books, 1995, p. 54.

Burch, Elizabeth, and Judith Sachs. *Natural Healing for the Pregnant Woman.* New York: Perigee, 1997, p. 74.

The Burton Goldberg Group. *Alternative Medicine: The Definitive Guide.* Puyallup, Wash.: Future Medicine Publishing, 1993.

"Drinking Has Effect on Fertility in Women." *Alcoholism & Drug Abuse Weekly*, v. 10 (35), September 14, 1998, p. 7.

Goldberg, Burton, and the Editors of *Alternative Medicine. Alternative Medicine Guide to Women's Health 1.* Tiburon, Calif.: Future Medicine Publishing, 1998, p. 166.

Lauersen, Niels H., and Colette Bouchez. *Getting Pregnant: What Couples Need to Know Right Now.* New York: Fawcett Columbine, 1991.

Northrup, Christiane. *Women's Bodies, Women's Wisdom: Creating Physical and Emotional Health and Healing.* New York: Bantam Books, 1998, p. 423.

Somer, Elizabeth. *Nutrition for a Healthy Pregnancy: The Complete Guide to Eating Before, During, and After Your Pregnancy.* New York: Henry Holt and Company, 1995.

Wesson, Nicki. *Enhancing Fertility Naturally: Holistic Therapies for a Successful Pregnancy.* Rochester, Vt.: Healing Arts Press, 1997, p. 71.

"Wine + Coffee = Infertility?" *Parents*, March 1999, p. 46.

Chapter 7   Herbal Therapy, Aromatherapy, Flower Remedies, and Other Natural Healing Systems

Bradstreet, Karen. *Overcoming Infertility Naturally: The Relationship Between Nutrition, Emotions and Reproduction.* Pleasant Grove, Utah: Woodland Books, 1995, p. 65.

The Burton Goldberg Group. *Alternative Medicine: The Definitive Guide.* Puyallup, Wash.: Future Medicine Publishing, 1993, pp. 54–55.

Conkling, Winifred. *Getting Pregnant Naturally: Healthy Choices to Boost Your Chances of Conceiving Without Fertility Drugs.* New York: Avon Books, 1999, pp. 71–72.

Green, Mindy, and Kathy Keville. *Aromatherapy: A Complete Guide to the Healing Art.* Freedom, Calif.: Crossing Press, 1995, "Therapeutics" chapter.

Ryman, Danielle. *Aromatherapy: The Complete Guide to Plant and Flower Essences for Health and Beauty.* New York: Bantam Books, 1993, pp. 15, 31.

Wesson, Nicki. *Enhancing Fertility Naturally: Holistic Therapies for a Successful Pregnancy.* Rochester, Vt.: Healing Arts Press, 1997, p. 121.

Chapter 8   Exercise, Movement Therapy, and Massage

The Burton Goldberg Group. *Alternative Medicine: The Definitive Guide.* Puyallup, Wash.: Future Medicine Publishing, 1993, pp. 427–428.

Northrup, Christiane. *Women's Bodies, Women's Wisdom: Creating Physical and Emotional Health and Healing.* New York: Bantam Books, 1998, p. 750.

Chapter 9   Breaking the Stress Cycle—Mind/Body Remedies for Relaxation

Domar, Alice D., and Henry Dreher. *Healing Mind, Healthy Woman: Using the Mind-Body Connection to Manage Stress and Take Control of Your Life.* New York: Henry Holt and Company, 1996, pp. 46–47.

Lark, Susan. *The Fibroid Tumors and Endometriosis Self-Help Book.* Berkeley, Calif.: Celestial Arts, 1995.

Payne, Niravi B., and Brenda Lane Richardson. *The Whole Person Fertility Program*SM: *A Revolutionary Mind-Body Process to Help You Conceive.* New York: Three Rivers Press, 1997, pp. xx–xxi.

Chapter 10   Keeping Your Sex Drive Active

Conkling, Winifred. *Getting Pregnant Naturally: Healthy Choices to Boost Your Chances of Conceiving Without Fertility Drugs.* New York: Avon Books, 1999, chapter 2.

Lauersen, Niels H., and Colette Bouchez. *Getting Pregnant: What Couples Need to Know Right Now.* New York: Fawcett Columbine, 1991, pp. 136–138, 202.

Haas, Elson M. *Staying Healthy with Nutrition: The Complete Guide to Diet and Nutritional Medicine.* Berkeley, Calif.: Celestial Arts, 1992, "Sexual Vitality" chapter.

Watson, Cynthia Mervis. *Love Potions: A Guide to Aphrodisiacs and Sexual Pleasures.* New York: Tarcher/Putnam, 1993, chapters 3, 4, and 7.

Resources

Fertility and Infertility

American College of Obstetricians and Gynecologists
P.O. Box 96920
409 Twelfth St., S.W.
Washington, DC 20090-6920
Phone: (202) 638-5577

American Society for Reproductive Medicine
1209 Montgomery Highway
Birmingham, AL 35216-2809
Phone: (205) 978-5000
E-mail: asrm@asrm.org
Web site: www.asrm.org

Fertility Research Foundation
1430 Second Ave., Ste. 103
New York, NY 10021
Phone: (212) 744-5500

Institute for Reproductive Health
Georgetown University
2115 Wisconsin Ave., Ste. 602
Washington, DC 20007
Phone: (202) 687-1392

International Council on Infertility Information
    Dissemination
P.O. Box 91363
Tucson, AZ 85721-5251
Phone: (520) 544-9548

National Infertility Network Exchange
P.O. Box 204
East Meadow, NY 11554
Phone: (516) 794-5772
E-mail: nine204@aol.com

Reproductive Toxicology Center
2440 M St., N.W., Ste. 217
Washington, DC 20037-1404
Phone: (202) 293-5137

RESOLVE
1310 Broadway
Somerville, MA 02144-1731
Phone: (617) 623-1156/623-0252 (help line)
Fax: (617) 623-0252
Web site: www.resolve.org

Pregnancy and Women's Health

Endometriosis Association
8585 N. 76th Place
Milwaukee, WI 53223
Phone: (800) 992-3636

International Childbirth Education Association
P.O. Box 20048
Minneapolis, MN 55420
Phone: (612) 854-8660

Menstrual Health Foundation
Womankind
P.O. Box 1775
Sebastopol, CA 95473
Phone: (707) 522-8662

National Women's Health Network
Phone: (212) 593-2141

Planned Parenthood Federation of America
810 Seventh Ave.
New York, NY 10019
Phone: (212) 541-7800
Web site: www.plannedparenthood.org

Alternative Medicine

American Association of Naturopathic Physicians
601 Valley St., Ste. 105
Seattle, WA 98109
Phone: (206) 298-0126
Web site: www.naturopathic.org

American Holistic Health Association
P.O. Box 17400
Anaheim, CA 92817-7400
Phone: (714) 779-6152
E-mail: ahha@healthy.net

American Holistic Medical Association
4101 Lake Boone Trail
Raleigh, NC 27607
Phone: (919) 787-5181

Holistic Health Directory and Resource Guide
42 Pleasant St.
Watertown, MA 02172
Phone: (617) 926-0200

World Research Foundation
20501 Ventura Blvd., Ste. 100
Woodland Hills, CA 91364
Phone: (818) 999-5483
Fax: (818) 227-6484

Acupuncture

American Association of Acupuncture and Oriental Medicine
433 Front St.
Catasauqua, PA 18032
Phone: (610) 266-1433

Council of Colleges of Acupuncture and Oriental Medicine
8403 Colesville Rd., Ste. 370
Silver Springs, MD 20910
Phone: (310) 608-9175
Web site: www.ccaom.org

Aromatherapy

American Alliance of Aroma Therapy
P.O. Box 750428
Petaluma, CA 94975-0428

American Aromatherapy Association
P.O. Box 3679
S. Pasadena, CA 91031

Aromatherapy Institute and Research
P.O. Box 1222
Fair Oaks, CA 95628
Phone: (916) 965-7546

National Association of Holistic Aromatherapy
P.O. Box 17622
Boulder, CO 80308-0622

Uttati International
400 S. Beverly Dr., Ste. 214
Beverly Hills, CA 90212
Phone: (310) 556-5717

Chi Gung

Health Action
19 E. Mission St., Ste. 102
Santa Barbara, CA 93101
Phone: (805) 682-3230

National Qi Gong Association
Phone: (888) 233-3655

Qi Gong Institute/East–West Academy of the Healing Arts
450 Sutter St., Ste. 916
San Francisco, CA 94108
Phone: (415) 788-2227

Diet and Nutritional Supplementation

American Academy of Nutrition
3408 Sausalito Dr.
Corona Del Mar, CA 92625
Phone: (800) 290-4226

Consumer Nutrition Hotline
Phone: (800) 366-1655

Corsello Centers for Nutritional Complementary Medicine
200 W. 67th St.
New York, NY 10019
Phone: (212) 399-0222

National Institute of Nutritional Education
1010 S. Joliet St. #107
Aurora, CO 80012
Phone: (303) 340-2054

Price Pottenger Nutrition Foundation
P.O. Box 2614
La Mesa, CA 91943-2614
Phone: (619) 574-7763

Flower Remedies

Beyond the Rainbow
Web site: www.rainbowcrystal.com

DaKara Kies Company
P.O. Box 82203
Kenmore, WA 98028
Phone: (800) 813-3877

Dr. Edward Bach Healing Society
644 Merrick Rd.
Lynbrook, NY 11563

Flower Essence Services
P.O. Box 1769
Nevada City, CA 95959
Phone: (800) 548-0075/(530) 265-0258

Flower Essence Society
P.O. Box 459
Nevada City, CA 95959
Phone: (800) 736-9222/(530) 265-9163
Web site: www.flowersociety.org

Herbal Medicine

American Herbalists Guild
P.O. Box 1683
Soquel, CA 95073
Phone: (408) 464-2441

Herb Research Foundation
1007 Pearl St., Ste. 200
Boulder, CO 80302
Phone: (303) 449-2265
Web site: www.herbs.org

Quality Life Herbs
P.O. Box 565
Yarmouth, ME 04096
Phone: (207) 842-4929
Fax: (207) 846-3168

Homeopathy

Homeopathic Educational Services
2124 Kittredge St.
Berkeley, CA 94704
Phone: (510) 649-0294
Web site: www.homeopathic.com

National Center for Homeopathy
801 N. Fairfax St., Ste. 306
Alexandria, VA 22314
Phone: (703) 548-7790

Massage/Body Work

Acupressure Institute of America
1533 Shattuck Ave.
Berkeley, CA 94709
Phone: (800) 442-2232/(510) 845-1059

American Massage Therapy Association
820 Davis St., Ste. 100
Evanston, IL 60201-4444
Phone: (708) 864-0123

Associated Bodywork & Massage Professionals
28677 Buffalo Park Rd.
Evergreen, CO 80439
Phone: (800) 458-2267

Esalen Institute
Highway 1
Big Sur, CA 93920
Phone: (831) 667-3000

International Rolf Institute
P.O. Box 1868
Boulder, CO 80306
Phone: (303) 449-5903

World Chiropractic Alliance
2950 N. Dobson Rd.
Chandler, AZ 85224
(800) 347-1011

Mind/Body Medicine

American Board of Hypnotherapy
16842 Von Karman Ave., Ste. 475
Irvine, CA 92606
Phone: (800) 872-9996

Center for Mind/Body Medicine
5225 Connecticut Ave., N.W., Ste. 414
Washington, DC 20015
Phone: (202) 966-7338

Mind/Body Health Sciences, Inc.
393 Dixon Rd.
Boulder, CO 80302
Phone: (303) 440-8460

Mind/Body Medical Institute
Deaconess Hospital
1 Deaconess Rd.
Boston, MA 02215
Phone: (617) 632-9525

Whole Person Fertility Program^{SM}
100 Remsen St.
Brooklyn, NY 11201
Phone: (800) 666-HEALTH/(718) 625-4802
E-mail: niravi@aol.com

Sexuality

American Association of Sex Educators, Counselors
   and Therapists
P.O. Box 238
Mount Vernon, IA 52314
Phone: (319) 895-8407
Web site: www.aasect.org

Eve's Garden
119 W. 57th St., Ste. 420
New York, NY 10019
Phone: (800) 848-3837/(212) 575-8651

Femme Productions (erotic videos)
Phone: (800) 456-LOVE

Good Vibrations (sex toys)
1210 Valencia St.
San Francisco, CA 94110

Love Potions, Inc. (aphrodisiacs)
530 Wilshire Blvd., Ste. 203
Santa Monica, CA 90401
Phone: (800) 208-9678

Sexuality Information and Education Council of the U.S.
130 W. 42nd St., Ste. 2500
New York, NY 10036
Phone: (212) 819-9770
Web site: www.siecus.org

The Sexuality Library (erotic videos)
Phone: (415) 974-8985

Sky Dancing Tantra
Right Hand Productions
P.O. Box 544
Mill Valley, CA 94942
Phone: (415) 388-0431

Xandria Collection
Dept. PB0193
P.O. Box 31039
San Francisco, CA 94131

Yoga

International Kundalini Yoga Teachers' Association
Phone: (505) 753-0423

Yoga Journal
2054 University Ave.
Berkeley, CA 94704

Yoga Research and Education Center
Phone: (707) 928-9898
Web site: www.yogaresearchcenter.org

Adoption

Adoptive Families of America
2309 Como Ave.
St. Paul, MN 55108
Phone: (800) 372-3300/(651) 645-9955
Web site: www.adoptivefam.org

National Adoption Information Clearinghouse
330 C St., S.W.
Washington, DC 20477
Phone: (888) 251-0075/(703) 352-3488
E-mail: naic@calib.com
Web site: www.calib.com/naic

National Council for Adoption
1930 17th St., N.W.
Washington, DC 20009
Phone: (202) 328-1200

Assisted Reproductive Technology and Surrogacy

Society for Assisted Reproductive Technology
1209 Montgomery Highway
Birmingham, AL 35216
Phone: (205) 978-5000
E-mail: asrm@asrm.org

Organization of Parents Through Surrogacy
P.O. Box 611
Gurnee, IL 60031
Phone: (847) 782-0224
E-mail: director@opts.com
Web site: www.opts.com

Index